beat
cancer

We dedicate this book to Sabire and Peter
for all their love and support, not just during the
writing but over the many years of our working lives.

Mustafa Djamgoz and Jane Plant

beat
cancer

The 10-step plan to help you
overcome and prevent cancer

PROF. MUSTAFA DJAMGOZ
& PROF. JANE PLANT

1 3 5 7 9 10 8 6 4 2

First published in 2014 by Vermilion, an imprint of Ebury Publishing
A Random House Group company

The Random House Group Limited Reg. No. 954009

Addresses for companies within the Random House Group can be found at
www.randomhouse.co.uk

The Random House Group Limited supports the Forest Stewardship
Council® (FSC®), the leading international forest-certification organisation.
Our books carrying the FSC label are printed on FSC®-certified paper. FSC is
the only forest-certification scheme supported by the leading environmental
organisations, including Greenpeace. Our paper procurement policy
can be found at www.randomhouse.co.uk/environment

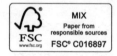

Designed and set by seagulls.net
Illustrations by Stephen Dew

Printed and bound in Great Britain by CPI Group (UK) Ltd, Croydon, CR0 4YY

ISBN 9780091947958

To buy books by your favourite authors and register for offers visit
www.randomhouse.co.uk

contents

foreword

This book is important and deserves to be taken seriously. It aims to empower all of us to cope better with cancer by providing us with the latest science written in accessible English. That means research that has been peer-reviewed and published in reputable international journals – in other words, the best. This book is the work of two eminent professors from Imperial College London, Mustafa Djamgoz, Professor of Cancer Biology, and Jane Plant, Professor of Geochemistry, who specialises in studying carcinogens such as arsenic in the environment. Jane has survived six episodes of breast cancer going back to 1987 when she was 42 years old. She is now almost 70 and is the picture of health with her cancer once again in remission.

The book is divided into ten steps designed to help you understand, prevent and manage cancer. The first step explains the exciting new findings about what cancer cells really are and what they do. In particular, it explains the increasingly important science of *epigenetics* and the *stem cell* characteristics of cancer. These are giving us new strategies to beat the disease and even to avoid it altogether. The rest of the book aims to help all of us (and I hope this includes medical professionals too) to develop an integrated approach to dealing with the disease. Hence it demonstrates how to combine the best conventional medical treatments to treat cancer with complementary therapies, exercise regimes and stress management to help healing in the longer term.

This is not a conventional cancer book. You will find many of the things you read illuminating; some of the information may be surprising and even, at times, shocking. However, all of the information is backed up by scientific research and fully referenced.

I recommend the book highly not only to cancer patients and their supporters but also to health professionals and administrators. Only by working together, with the patient as an integral part of the team, will real progress be made. I hope they will read the book and take on board its key messages to help us all to beat cancer.

Professor Sir Graeme Catto, MD, FRCP, FRSE
President, College of Medicine
Former President, General Medical Council
and Vice Principal, King's College London.

welcome

You may be looking at this book because you or someone you love has been diagnosed with cancer and you want to do everything possible to regain control of your health and life or that of your loved one. This book is designed to help you do just that. It should also be helpful for those who do not have the disease but wish to ensure that they do everything possible to reduce their risk of cancer, especially if they are in a high-risk group such as those with a family history of the disease. We want to help you to understand what cancer is, how it can be prevented and treated, and what you can do to help yourself. We want to help you to avoid developing cancer and, for those who already have the condition, to make sure that your medical treatment has the best possible chance of success. We aim to give you the best information based on the latest peer-reviewed scientific and medical literature and make it easily accessible to everyone.

The book is important because cancer is now a global problem and very much a part of modern life. In the West, our lifetime risk of developing it is now more than one in three and rising.[1] There can be few of us who have not been touched by the disease in some way – if not personally, then among our family and friends.

One point is especially important. Being diagnosed with cancer is no longer an inevitable death sentence. Many cancers can be treated. But treatment is not just about what the doctors do *to* you. It is also about how you work *with* your doctors – and how *they* work with you. Making sure your body is as fit as possible can make a real difference in fighting the condition. We aim to help those diagnosed with cancer to put their disease into remission using changes in diet and lifestyle, in combination with conventional treatment.

the story of this book

This book sprang from our joint desire to enable people affected by, or at risk of, cancer to do everything possible to protect themselves. Mustafa and Jane are experienced scientists working on cancer biology and environmental pollutants, respectively, at Imperial College London, one of the most highly rated universities in the world. Much of Mustafa's work is concerned with developing new and innovative treatments that could prevent cancer cells from spreading through the body. Such treatments have the potential to enable patients even with advanced cancer to live with their disease, in the same way that people live with diabetes, asthma and other chronic diseases. Jane is an international authority on hazardous substances, especially carcinogens (cancer-causing substances) such as arsenic,[2] radioactive elements and hormone-disrupting chemicals found in pharmaceuticals, plasticisers, pesticides and detergents.[3] Her research is aimed at reducing their risk to human health. Until recently, she chaired the UK Government's Advisory Committee on Hazardous Substances. Jane also has a very personal interest in cancer prevention as she has, against all the odds, overcome breast cancer an incredible six times in the last 28 years.

Jane's story of defeating breast cancer

Jane first developed breast cancer in 1987. She had a mastectomy, but the cancer returned four times over the next five years, each time spreading to lymph nodes near the original cancer. In 1993, with a secondary cancer the size of an egg in her neck, she was told the chemotherapy was not working and she had only two months to live. That was horrific news. Jane was just as frightened as any of us would be, but as a scientist her immediate instinct was to research to find out why she had contracted cancer and what she could do to help herself. She and her husband had worked in China and knew that Chinese women there had very low rates of breast cancer at that time. They discovered that breast cancer was also rare in other oriental countries such as Japan and Thailand. Yet women from these places appeared to be at just as much risk as American or European women when they moved to the West. The only differences seemed to be diet and lifestyle. We will tell you more about what Jane discovered later in this book and how her work with Mustafa is providing clear guidelines underpinned by sound science to help beat cancer.

Jane changed to an Asian-type diet overnight. That seemed to allow the chemotherapy to kick in. Within days, her cancer was shrinking and within six weeks, there was no sign of it. Until 2011 she had remained free of the disease for almost 20 years and had published her story and findings in her international bestselling book *Your Life in Your Hands*.[4]

In December 2011, however, she was diagnosed again with breast cancer. At the time, she had a large lump beneath her collar bone which had spread over an area of 80 cm^2, another secondary tumour in the lining of her right lung, and small secondary tumours throughout her right lung. She realised just how lax she had become about her diet and lifestyle. She returned immediately to her Asian-type[5] diet with a daily exercise routine and used meditation and other stress-management techniques in combination with the tiny dose of letrozole prescribed by her oncologist. After only three weeks the fluid had cleared from her lung and the lump beneath her collar bone had reduced to an area of less than 36 cm^2. By July Jane was told once again that her cancer was in remission.

Jane has lived nearly half her adult life with breast cancer. It was her personal experience that led her to undertake research into the disease alongside her day job and she is convinced that an approach that integrates the best of conventional medicine with a good diet and lifestyle is essential to beating cancer. She has written a number of books about cancer[6] for the general reader and runs a website, www.cancersupportinternational.com, which carries useful information about cancer.

Mustafa's research – neuroscience solutions to cancer!

Mustafa trained in neuroscience and studied the workings of the brain for some 25 years before becoming interested in cancer! He is the first to investigate systematically electrical signals in cancer cells and has discovered that, in order to spread, cancer cells become electrically excitable and hyperactive, rather like nerve cells in an out-of-control epileptic brain. He is now involved in developing new and innovative treatments based on that research and already a new drug is in preparation for clinical trial. The primary aim of his research is to control cancer non-toxically, that is without chemotherapy! He has also established a small charity, Pro-Cancer Research Fund (PCRF) that supports the new research and runs the Amber Care Centre, a drop-in facility in north London for cancer patients and their families.

Jane and Mustafa were introduced to each other about 10 years ago by a colleague at Imperial. As Jane learnt more and more about Mustafa's research, he developed an interest in Jane's work on carcinogens in the environment and her research into the role of dietary and lifestyle factors. We have thus come to the study of cancer from different directions – Mustafa from the background of a lab-based scientist and Jane from field and laboratory work in many countries trying to identify links between the environment and human health. It is remarkable how, from these different directions, we have reached very similar conclusions. Cancer is not just bad luck: we know more about its causes than ever before. For many sufferers, it no longer needs to be a death sentence. Even in the case of aggressive metastatic cancer we now know the sequence of events involved. Already, a lot can be done to prevent and treat cancer, at least to the point where we can live with it, as the increasing survival rates demonstrate. For instance, more than three-quarters of women diagnosed with breast cancer now survive for 10 years or more. In the 1970s, just 44 per cent survived for this length of time.[7] There has been a similar increase in survival rates for men with prostate cancer. This may be linked to better testing, enabling the disease to be identified at an earlier stage. Understanding the processes involved in the development and spread of cancer explains why Jane's approach to complementing her medical treatment with a change in lifestyle and diet works and why she is still here 25 years after her first diagnosis of breast cancer.

We both understand just how daunting a cancer diagnosis can be and how hard the process of treatment and recovery can be. In addition to carrying out our research, we both work through our own charities, websites and other organisations to help cancer patients personally. We understand the humanity needed to help people to deal with this most dreaded of diseases and to put it into remission.

This book brings together our expertise to give you the best possible evidence-based advice.

There is a great deal we can do for ourselves in our everyday lives, both to avoid the disease and to support medical treatment in helping our bodies to fight it. The book explains the latest scientific thinking, building on evidence from the work of distinguished international scientists. Some of the ideas are yet to be accepted widely, but they are based on impeccable science. Not surprisingly, you will come across words and concepts you may not be familiar with. We aim to explain these clearly as they occur. More than anything, though, the book is the product of Jane's and Mustafa's many discussions with each other – and with their brilliant students.

how to use the book

Clinical medicine is necessarily conservative! It takes a long time for new ideas to be accepted. Even when adopted, clinical trials may take many months before evidence emerges and new drugs or procedures enter clinical practice. Increasingly, however, cancer-support centres such as the Maggie's Cancer Caring Centres in our major hospitals are using a more integrated approach to cancer treatment. Throughout this book, we have adopted an integrated evidence-based approach to preventing and treating cancer, combining conventional treatment with the best complementary therapies such as diet and exercise. The information and advice we give are based predominantly on peer-reviewed publications, and each of the chapters in the book has been critically assessed by two or more experts in the field. In any case, the whole of our stance is derived from sound established scientific principles. References are given throughout the book, so it is possible to go deeper into the various topics being covered, should you or your doctors wish.

This book is divided into 10 chapters, each representing one step on the path to living a healthy life – ideally without cancer! To have any chance of preventing cancer or beating it and keeping it in remission, we need to understand what cancer is, how it develops and progresses, what treatments are available and how we can make sure our bodies are in the best possible state to combat it. The first of our 10 steps is a modern, rational, scientific explanation of what cancer is, and we then take you through all aspects of conventional treatments, complementary therapies and dietary and lifestyle factors. We hope you will find the steps helpful in beating or controlling the disease or – even better – avoiding it. Each chapter or step is written as a stand-alone and can be read on its own. Or you may wish to read the whole book through to learn all about the best ways to beat the disease. The book includes science facts in boxes, which some readers may wish to skip or come back to later. However you choose to use the book, we wish you well on your mission to understand and beat cancer.

step 1
inform yourself

If you or a loved one has been diagnosed with cancer, or even if you simply want to do all you can to avoid it, your first step is to understand what cancer is and how you can help your body fight it. The knowledge you gain here will help you to take action to reduce your risk. If you already have a diagnosis, you will be better able to understand what your doctors tell you, know what questions to ask and then decide, with them, on the choice of treatments to ensure the best possible outcome.

Although cancer is a complex disease modern research is rapidly revealing its secrets. It was not so long ago that the stigma attached to the 'C word' or the 'big C' meant that people would talk about it in hushed tones behind closed doors. Thankfully times have changed – and so has the outlook for people with cancer. Cancer is no longer the inevitable killer it once was. Although between a third and half of us will develop cancer at some time in our lives, our chances of survival are better than ever, particularly when cancer is diagnosed early. And the good news is that prevention is fast becoming a reality. What we hope to do in this book is explain what you can do in your everyday life to boost your odds of beating cancer.

about cancer

Cancer is not a single disease. There are more than two hundred different types of cancer that can affect various parts of the body.

Even cancers of specific organs, like breast or lung, may include several different subtypes, which behave differently and need different treatments. Breast cancers, for example, can develop in different parts of the breast. In some, the cancer's growth is driven by hormones, while in others it is not. Cancers also vary in their biochemical properties and in how quickly they may grow and spread. Hardly surprising then that there is no single treatment or therapy that works for all cancers or even cancers of individual organs.

Doctors will never say that cancer is cured; only that it is in *remission*. If even a single cell remains after treatment, it can replicate and start the cancer growing again. For that reason, cancer is now regarded by many doctors as a chronic disease, much like diabetes or asthma.[1]

Cancer types

Cancers are often grouped by the tissue where they originated. You may come across these names if you or someone you know has a diagnosis.

- *Carcinomas* develop in the tissues that cover external and internal body surfaces and are made up of what are called *epithelial* cells. Carcinomas are the most common cancers and include lung, breast and colon (or bowel) cancer.
- *Sarcomas* begin in the cells of the supportive tissues in the body, such as bone, connective tissue, muscle, fat and cartilage.
- *Lymphomas* develop in the lymph nodes and the body's immune system.
- *Leukaemias* develop in blood cells in the bone marrow and tend to be found in large numbers in the blood.

Age matters

Every year, more than 300,000 people in the UK develop cancer for the first time[2] – three-quarters of them in people aged 60 or over and one-third in the over 75s. Only one in 10 are diagnosed in people aged 25–49. The risk of most cancers increases with age as your body experiences wear and tear and is bombarded by undesirable environmental factors. A small number of cancers affect children, notably some leukaemias, but childhood cancer is thankfully rare with around only 1,500 new cases each year in the UK.[3]

Cancer and culture

Although cancer affects people the world over, there are dramatic differences between the types of cancer common in the richer West – Europe, including the UK, and USA – and those which are more likely to affect people in developing countries. The affluent West and developing nations are poles apart in cancer, as in so much else. The difference is so stark that we now refer to cancers of affluence and cancers of poverty (see Figure 1.1, page 18).[4]

We can learn a lot from these differences and by studying different communities with markedly different diets and cultures. In the West, for example, hormone-related cancers such as breast and prostate are among the most common. But in poorer countries, cancers caused by infection – stomach, liver and cervical cancers – are far more prevalent. The proportion of cancers caused by viruses is three times greater in East Asia than it is in the UK, and even higher in many African countries, yet hormone-related cancers are less common, even in relatively rich countries like Japan. Ever since reliable cancer registries began to be kept in the 1950s, we have seen a dramatic difference between oriental and Western countries in the numbers affected by breast and prostate cancer. The incidence

A. Breast

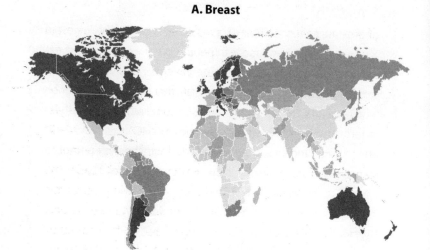

Age-standardised incidence rates per 100,000

B. Liver

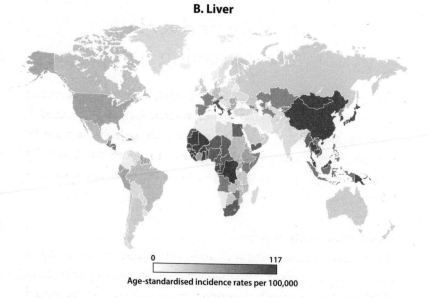

Age-standardised incidence rates per 100,000

Figure 1.1 *Breast (A) and liver (B) cancers as examples of cancers of affluence and poverty, respectively. The darker the shading, the higher the incidence.*

of prostate cancer in Japan, for instance, is one of the lowest in the world. Yet when Japanese people live in the West and eat a Western diet, their risk of these cancers rapidly rises to the same level as the locals. That suggests that the cause cannot be wholly genetic or hereditary, it must also be related to lifestyle. In fact, the World Health Organisation (WHO) say that 30–40 per cent of cancers can be prevented if we change our diet to something more like that in many Eastern countries.[5] Sadly, the spread of the Western diet and lifestyle is having a dramatic impact on cancer rates. The latest data from the International Agency for Research on Cancer shows that Eastern countries are rapidly catching up with the West. We shall talk in more detail about the role of diet and lifestyle in Steps 5, 6, 7 and 8.

why cancer develops – cells behaving badly

Cancer is not a new disease. In fact, Hippocrates first described and named it 2,500 years ago in ancient Greece. He called it *karkinos,* the ancient Greek word for crab, perhaps because he thought cancer was an alien organism invading the body. We now know that is wrong. Cancer is in fact just our own cells behaving badly.[6]

How your body works

All the tissues and structures within our bodies are made up of more than 100 trillion (100 followed by 12 zeros) tiny cells, most of which are constantly reproducing themselves (or we would simply wear out). Different tissues are made up of different types of specialised cells. For instance, white blood cells are different from red blood cells, and both are different from bone or muscle cells. Many tissues also contain specialised stem cells which are important for the growth of our tissues as we mature, as well as for tissue regeneration following injury or damage. During wound healing, for example, skin cells and skin stem cells multiply to repair the damage and move to close the gap. In a healthy body, biochemical signals instruct cells when to start and stop growing or tell them they should move or stop so that tissues and organs can be repaired as necessary and stay in good shape.

When things go wrong

Cancer happens when something goes wrong with the systems that regulate these processes so that cells lose control and start multiplying in an uncontrolled way. When this happens it results in a lump which may be benign or cancerous. Benign lumps are different to cancers – they normally grow slowly, do not spread and only cause problems if they grow very large or put pressure on the tissue where they are growing.

If the cells are cancerous they can also invade the surrounding healthy tissue – known as 'local spread' – and can spread to other more distant parts of the body – a process known as 'metastasis'. If, for example, breast cancer spreads to the lungs, the cancer cells are still breast cancer cells, not lung cancer. It is this ability to spread that makes cancer so dangerous – in fact most cancer deaths result from metastatic disease, not the original (primary) tumour. That is why screening and early diagnosis are both so important.

What makes cancer cells different?

Although there are many different types of cancer, their cells have certain common characteristics that set them apart from normal cells. Cancer researchers Douglas Hanahan and Robert Weinberg defined the 'hallmarks of cancer',[7, 8] which show just how different they are to normal cells (see table opposite).

Normal cells	Cancer cells
Only divide when signalled to do so by the body's biochemical control system. Another signal tells them when to stop dividing.	Keep growing and multiplying in an uncontrolled way because of signalling abnormalities and ignore instructions that tell them to stop.
When cells are damaged a molecular brake halts cell division until they are repaired. If they are damaged beyond repair, they are programmed to die (apoptosis) so damaged cells which could harm nearby healthy cells are eliminated.	The molecular brake does not work and they lack the mechanism that triggers the process of apoptosis.
Can divide only a limited number of times (50–70) before they wear out and die.	Can keep dividing indefinitely.
They are inactivated when they touch each other (known as 'contact inhibition').	They remain active and keep reproducing despite contact with other cells around them.
Metabolise glucose to produce energy in the mitochondria using oxygen.	Metabolise glucose anaerobically (without oxygen) in the main body of the cell and consume far more glucose than normal cells.
Do not travel – e.g. breast cells stay in the breast, lung cells stay in the lung.	Can travel via the blood stream and lymphatic system to other parts of the body where they can develop secondary tumours.

Angiogenesis

Oxygen is essential for the survival of all cells, but once a growing tumour reaches a size of 0.5–1 millimetre, it becomes too big for oxygen to diffuse into it from existing blood vessels. *Angiogenesis* is the ability of cancer cells to create and attract new blood vessels, so that they can obtain a continuous supply of oxygen and other nutrients and eliminate the waste products generated during their growth.

Why doesn't our immune system destroy cancer cells?

Our immune system quite simply is not efficient in detecting cancer because tumours consist of our own (albeit damaged) cells. This also makes developing cancer vaccines difficult. However, vaccines have been developed against at least some cancer-causing viruses such as the human papilloma virus which is associated with cervical cancer.

How the lymphatic system works

As your blood circulates, a colourless fluid (*lymph*) leaks out of the capillaries into tissues before draining into fine *lymph vessels*. Lymph contains large numbers of several types of white blood cells called *lymphocytes*, which are important in fighting disease. Lymph generally moves around the body more slowly than blood because it is not pumped around by the heart.

The small lymph vessels join together to form larger tubes which pass through *lymph glands* (or *nodes*) in various parts of the body including the armpits, neck, groin and abdomen. They vary from the size of a pinhead to that of a baked bean, and their number varies from person to person; there are usually between 15 and 30 in the armpit, for instance. These lymph nodes trap and try to destroy anything harmful, such as bacteria and viruses. Sometimes they cannot do this immediately, and the lymph nodes swell and become painful in response to the infection. The immune system includes specialist organs such as the tonsils, adenoids, spleen and thymus which have important roles in fighting disease.

The lymphatic system also provides a route – along with blood vessels – for cancer cells to spread. A type of cancer called *lymphoma* originates in the lymph nodes themselves; they swell, but are usually painless. There are many other reasons for such symptoms, but if you can feel painless but swollen lymph glands, it is important to have them checked by your doctor.

how cancer develops

'Solid' tumours that develop as lumps of cancer cells like breast or bowel cancer (as opposed to 'non-solid' cancers of the blood – leukaemias) have three main stages of development (see Figure 1.2, below).[9]

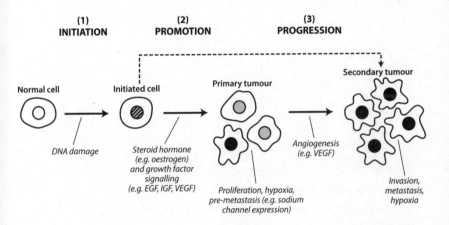

Figure 1.2 *The three main stages of cancer.*

- *Initiation* – when the DNA (deoxyribonucleic acid) of the genes that control cell reproduction (known as 'cell-cycle genes') is damaged, for example by environmental factors such as ionising radiation or tobacco smoke.
- *Promotion* – when initiated cells multiply to form a collection of cancer cells – 'primary tumour'.
- *Progression* – when the primary tumour develops further and starts to spread, initially locally and then through the body – metastasis.

However, it is possible in some cancers, especially aggressive ones, to go direct from initiation to progression.

The promotion of initiated cancer cells

the promotion stage is when the primary tumour has started growing and cancer cells are multiplying. In some cancers, notably cancers of the blood, there is no solid tumour, just large numbers of circulating cancer cells. Scientists believe that what happens at the promotion stage is crucial in determining whether the earliest cancer cells – the initiated cells – survive and go on to become a tumour. The process is rather like watering and fertilising (initiated) cancer 'seeds'[10] or providing oxygen to (initiated) cancer 'sparks'.[11] Increasingly research is linking cancer promotion to the presence of high levels of proteins called growth factors circulating in the body and, with hormone-dependent cancers, to high levels of hormones such as oestrogen and testosterone. As we will learn later in this chapter both growth factors and hormones normally act as chemical messengers in the body but they can promote cancer if their levels are out of balance. By changing the body's biochemistry, therefore, diet can impact upon hormones, growth factors and hence cancer (see Step 5).

How cancer spreads

We have learnt that cancer is the uncontrolled growth of cells and tissues. It can occur in almost any part of the body, but as long as it stays in the place where it developed it remains a primary tumour that can usually be removed by surgery and poses no further danger. It is cancers that spread to other parts of the body and cause secondary tumours (metastases) that are the most dangerous.

So how does this happen?

We used to think that cells in the primary tumour had to develop the ability to spread, and that this happened as they kept dividing and repeating the mistakes that had initially caused the cancer. But the recent discovery that a cell that has just become cancerous may *already* have the gene combination it needs to metastasise has challenged this view. In fact, we now know that sometimes metastatic disease occurs without a primary tumour being clinically identifiable. A common example of this is the smoking-related small-cell lung cancer.

Metastasis

Once they are able to spread, some cancer cells detach from each other, break off from the tissue where they are growing and ultimately enter the body's circulation system. Where the primary tumour is very close to the circulatory system they can enter directly – breast cancer, for example, spreads mechanically first to the under-arm lymph glands, which are close to the breast ducts where most breast cancers arise.

Alternatively, cancer cells can enter blood vessels – a process called *intravasation* where the cancer cells have to squeeze through tight spaces in the blood vessel wall. Once in the circulation system, they can survive for months, even years. Many of them will die – killed off by the white blood cells or battered by the fast flowing blood – it has been estimated that only one in every 10,000 cancer cells entering the blood circulation ultimately survives. That's the good news. But if even a few cells survive and reach their target they can squeeze back through a blood vessel wall (extravasation) into the tissue of any organ close by. Different cancer cells tend to lodge at different organs – for example, breast and prostate cancer often spread to bone. Once they find the right environment the cells can settle, start multiplying again and form secondary tumours.

However, not all these extravasating cancer cells go on to form full-blown secondary tumours. Quite often, they form only 'micro-metastases' – too tiny to be detected, even on a scan – which can remain dormant for years. In essence, they remain in hibernation, possibly because of signals they receive from the primary tumour that prevent them developing a supply of new blood vessels that would enable them to grow – known as angiogenesis.[12]

The primary tumour can send out signals that either promote the formation of new blood vessels or inhibit it. It appears that some primary tumours may stop secondary tumours from fully developing by releasing inhibitory signals. This is rather like the behaviour of a parasite which wants to keep its host alive for as long as possible.[13]

This is crucial when it comes to treatment. The oncologist must always take account of the fact that there may be micro-metastases when deciding on the best treatment. It also means that it is not always the best thing to operate and remove the primary tumour as this could be sending out inhibitory signals and removing it may clear the way for micro-metastases to grow and form secondary tumours. All this reinforces our view that cancer is best managed by research-active clinicians practising in teaching or specialist hospitals or with links to such hospitals (see Step 3).

our new understanding

So what triggers cells to become cancerous and grow? The latest research suggests that much of the answer lies in *stem cells*.

The role of stem cells

We have seen that cancer develops when the signals that regulate how cells divide and multiply go wrong, and there is increasing evidence that this involves stem cells.

Stem cells are the body's raw materials – the cells from which all other cells with specialised functions are formed. Embryonic stem cells, the cells found in the very earliest stages of the embryo, are able to become any type of body cell – this is how the embryo develops into a baby. As the embryonic stem cell keeps reproducing, its daughter cells ultimately become heart, brain, bone and many other types of cell. These remarkable embryonic stem cells disappear within a few days of birth. Adult stem cells are found in small numbers in most adult tissues and have a more limited repertoire than embryonic stem cells, linked to the tissue or organ where they are situated. Like regular cells, these specialised stem cells divide to form two identical new cells – so a breast stem cell will divide to produce two breast stem cells, unlike embryonic stem cells, which have the remarkable ability to transform into different cell types. Remarkably, this process may be reversible, at least to some extent, and a recent (2014) paper published in the world-famous journal *Nature* has shown that mature cells may be forced to acquire stemness by being shocked in acid.[14]

What appears to happen as cancer grows is that distorted signals cause some of the new cells created from cell division to switch back into something like their neonatal or embryonic stem-cell form, instead of their specialised adult form.*

Another characteristic of embryonic stem cells is that they are capable of dividing and renewing themselves for long periods – far longer than ordinary cells which eventually age and die – so they are able to increase their numbers very rapidly. Cancer cells seem to behave in a similar way, so the obvious question is: do embryonic stem cells have a role in the development of cancer?

Scientists argued for more than 10 years about whether cancer stem cells actually exist and, if they do, whether they drive the development of cancer. It was one of the biggest scientific controversies in cancer research. Now three separate studies on mice, all published in 2012, have resolved it.[15] Three groups, working independently – in the USA, Belgium and the Netherlands – looked at brain, skin and intestinal cancers, respectively, and all

---

* Cancer cells appear to flip back to have embryonic stem-cell-like characteristics. The technical term for such cells is neonatal because they usually disappear within days after the birth of a baby animal or human.

found direct evidence of stem cells driving cancer growth. The suggestion is that the same is true of all cancers that produce solid tumours.

What this means for cancer treatment

The similarities between cancer stem cells and healthy embryonic stem cells have important implications for treatment. Any therapy that targets cancer stem cells may also attack healthy tissues and cause widespread damage. But if researchers can identify significant differences between normal adult cells and cancer stem cells they may be able to develop therapies that distinguish between them, and target only cancer stem cells, leaving healthy cells untouched.

Like embryonic stem cells, cancer cells have an extraordinary ability to transform themselves. This means that treatments like chemotherapy, which are aimed at killing them, may actually encourage the development of drug-resistant cells which survive treatment and form a new cancer (Figure 1.3, below). What this

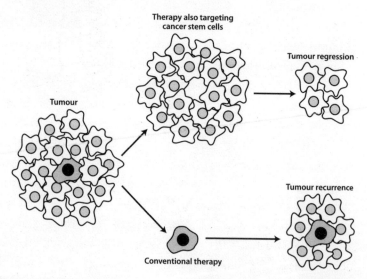

Figure 1.3 *Comparison of conventional chemotherapy with treatment which also target stem cells. Tumour regression is more likely with the latter.*

means for patients is that, in some cases, aggressive chemotherapy aimed at destroying the cancer may not be the best treatment. In fact, it may be better to control the cancer and stop it from proliferating and spreading rather than trying to kill it outright.

How good cells turn bad

We have looked at what happens to individual body cells, but now we need to go deeper and discover what happens at the genetic level to change healthy cells into dangerous cancer cells.

DNA provides the basic code for all life on earth. It is the substance that our genes are made of and it produces the proteins in our bodies that carry out all the activities that keep us alive. Our genes are strung out along chromosomes which are found in the nucleus of every cell in our body, except red blood cells which lack a nucleus (Figure 1.4, below).

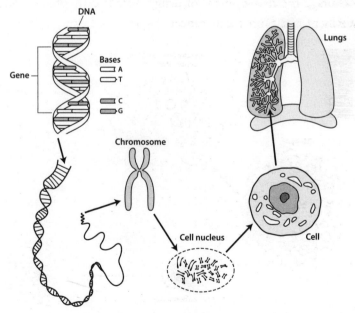

Figure 1.4 *The relationship between DNA, genes and chromosomes which are in the cell nuclei of all the tissues that make up our organs, such as lungs.*

Humans have 23 pairs of chromosomes: one of each pair is inherited from our mother, the other from our father. You might inherit the gene for brown hair from your mother and red hair from your father, in which case your hair will be brown because that gene is dominant. Together, our genes contain all the information that makes us what we are: everything from the colour of our eyes to whether we are right-handed or left-handed – and whether or not we have a predisposition to develop a particular disease, including a type of cancer.

After Crick and Watson discovered the structure of DNA – the famous double helix – and after its sequencing, scientists believed that our genetic inheritance was the only thing that mattered in terms of our make-up and risk of disease. Indeed until the completion of the Human Genome Project in 2003 when scientists had identified and mapped all our genes, it was believed that we had more than 100,000 genes.[16] Astonishingly, the actual number turned out to be only around 22,000 – far fewer than expected. What's more, as research continued more amazing facts emerged. A study published in 2011 showed that the genome of a simple water flea called *Daphnia* – a creature about two millimetres long – has about 31,000 genes, approximately 50 per cent more than us.[17] A banana has 36,000 genes! How on earth could that be? The answer lies in the fact that 98 per cent of our DNA does not consist of real 'genes' but of regulatory material (once called 'junk DNA') that determines how – and to what extent – our various genes are *'expressed'*, in other words how the information from each gene is used.

A powerful example of the impact of gene expression is the caterpillar and the butterfly.[18] Both have exactly the same set of genes. In the larval stage, the pattern of gene expression forms a caterpillar. But then in the adult, following pupation, different organisation of the same genes results in changed form which produces a beautiful butterfly. If differences in the expression of the same set of genes can give such extraordinarily diverse results as the caterpillar and the butterfly, it is easy to see that the processes that control gene expression play a crucial role in determining our form and function.

The new science of epigenetics

The water flea *Daphnia* has large numbers of genes whose function is fixed and virtually no regulatory material. We, on the other hand, are dependent on the regulation of the expression levels and patterns of our genes to generate our vastly diverse bodily functions. The new and rapidly growing science of *epigenetics*, which literally means *beyond* or *around genetics*, is the study of how genes 'behave' and are regulated, including by being influenced by the environment. All this has important things to teach us about cancer. Epigenetics means that our genes are not fixed and, as such, do not necessarily determine our fate. It is certainly true that if we are blue-eyed we are not suddenly going to become brown-eyed, but a large number of genes are *malleable*. The way the particular function of each manifests itself can vary according to the conditions affecting the cell. What's more, the genes of a given cell may not all be 'switched on' all the time. Many genes sit quietly, doing nothing very much, until their particular function is needed or until something happens in the body to switch them on.

One way to think of it is to imagine genes as a string of lights. We used to think that cancer happened when one or more lights in a given string were damaged or when something went wrong with the order they were arranged in: their sequence. What epigenetics now tells us is that some of the lights can be turned up (up-regulated genes) or turned down (down-regulated genes), switched on or switched off, or perhaps have shades over them dampening down gene expression. It is the inherent malleability of human genes that explains both the sophistication of the human body and our susceptibility to *epigenetic* diseases, including cancer.

Cancer and genes

We know that cancer happens when something goes wrong with the genes that control cell division and multiplication, known as the cell-cycle genes. These are the *proto-oncogenes*, 'grow genes',[19] which, if they go wrong, can turn into *oncogenes* and act as a kind of accelerator on cell replication.

The *tumour-suppressor genes*, or 'don't grow genes' normally act as a brake to stop cell replication. If they are damaged or mutated, however, the brake fails and may allow cells to grow out of control. Some types of tumour-suppressor genes can also fix breaks and repair damage to DNA.

The *apoptotic genes*, such as the p53 gene (see also page 37), which are sometimes grouped with tumour-suppressor genes, normally operate from the cell nucleus by inducing repair or, if that is not possible, instructing the cell to commit suicide, apoptosis.

The role of one group of tumour-suppressor genes known as 'gatekeepers' has been emphasised by recent epigenetic studies. There is evidence that when these genes are 'silenced' the cell loses many of its specialised characteristics, becoming more like an undifferentiated embryonic stem cell. Silencing of such tumour-suppressor genes is thought to lock the cells into a perpetual state of self-renewal, which makes them predisposed to become cancerous.[20]

Thanks to epigenetics we now know that cancer depends not just on individual genes, but on the interaction between our genes and their surroundings, determined by our lifestyle and environmental factors which can cause damage and/or alter gene expression.[21] So even if you have cancer-causing genes, they may not become active until and unless particular conditions arise that switch them on – and if the conditions change, they might be switched off. That was demonstrated in a stunning trial published in 2005 with men who had a firm diagnosis of early-stage prostate cancer but had opted for a 'wait and see' approach rather than immediate treatment.[22] The study found that, at least at this early stage, cancer-causing genes can be switched off and protective genes switched on simply by changes in diet and lifestyle – and that this actually inhibited the growth of tumours, just within a few months. It was followed by another pilot study in 2008, which found that 453 of the genes associated with prostate cancer had been switched off and 48 protective genes had been switched on.[23] Later in the book, we will look at what might trigger cancer-causing genes – and protective genes – to switch on and off.

When the dominoes fall

The way that cancer develops is rather like the game of domino toppling. The intricate line of dominoes standing on end and arranged in complicated curves and branches represents your body's normal, disease-free state. When cancer strikes, it pushes the first domino over and all the rest topple in order.

The first domino to topple may be the 'gatekeeper' tumour-suppressor genes, that are involved in keeping the cell in its specialised adult form. If these are silenced or put out of action, the first domino falls. Then other genes are free to flip back to their embryonic form – and more dominoes topple over.

Two important sets of genes that appear to flip back to their embryonic form and are important in the progression of cancer are the genes controlling cell metabolism and the channel that allows sodium into cells and affects their electrical 'excitability'. In cancer cells lack of oxygen (hypoxia) both accompanies and promotes the changed activity of the sodium channel. When cancer cells become hypoxic they form lactic acid, which is toxic so they need to excrete it. This in turn leads to the development of an acid 'envelope' around the cancer cells which activates digestive enzymes which degrade the cells' surroundings clearing the way for these aggressive cells to advance and metastasise (Figure 1.5). All these are crucial stages in the domino chain and this understanding offers promising routes to new treatments.[24]

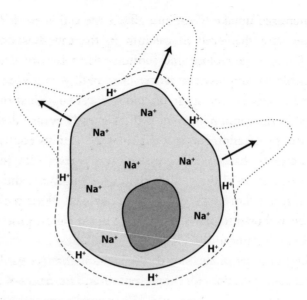

Figure 1.5 *A cancer cell showing its high level of internal sodium (Na⁺). This leads to acidification (H⁺) of the surrounding space which facilitates the invasiveness of the cancer cell (arrows).*

Excitable cancer cells

New research at Imperial College London and elsewhere has shown that aggressive cancer cells – those capable of metastasising – are electrically excitable[25] and it is this that makes them hyperactive, invasive and able to spread to distant organs (see pages 25–26). Thus, aggressive cancer cells behave rather like nerve cells in a state of seizure in an epileptic brain, with the body out of control in convulsions. This cell excitability has been shown in breast, prostate, lung, cervix, ovary and colon cancer and is probably a feature of all solid tumours.

Cancer cells become more excitable because the increase in the sodium channel together with the reduction in oxygen allows in more sodium, which increases electrical activity. At the same time, potassium, which by contrast has a calming effect on the cells is blocked which increases the excitation further.

Inherited cancer genes

Most cancers are caused by interactions between our genes and lifestyle factors that happen during our lifetimes, but some cancer genes are inherited. The faulty inherited breast cancer genes BRCA-1 and BRCA-2, which dramatically increase the risk of developing breast cancer, are probably the best known. The risk of disease is so high that some women with these faulty genes opt for a double mastectomy to prevent cancer developing. Although it sounds as if this type of cancer is a genetic disease it is more complicated than that. Although women who carry one of these genes certainly are at very high risk of developing breast cancer, they are not born with it and it takes many years before other changes occur and the disease develops. So while there are genes which increase your predisposition to certain cancers, cancer is not inherited in the same way as colour blindness or diseases like cystic fibrosis.

Some other cancer-causing genes have also been identified. Most involve mutations of the tumour-suppressor genes. A gene called p53, for example, produces a protein capable of halting the whole cell cycle until DNA damage is repaired or cell suicide is triggered. Damage to p53 is regarded as a key factor in a number of cancers. There are many others, and almost certainly more yet to be discovered. At present, we can test for some of these damaged genes but not all.

Cancer promoters

Growth factors and hormones act as chemical messengers with a particular set of instructions, and exert a powerful influence on the body, regulating many essential body processes. They may play a key role in creating the conditions that cause the dominoes to start falling in the long, complicated collapse that leads to cancer – for example by driving an increase in the expression of the sodium channel (see pages 33–35).

Hormones

Hormones make things happen – the word comes from the Greek word *hormein*, to excite. They have many different functions in the body, helping to regulate metabolism, immune functions, salt-and-water balance and much more. The steroid hormones like oestrogens, progestogens and androgens are fat-soluble, which means they can pass through the cell membrane. Because they can get right inside the cell, they are also able to change gene expression. Non-steroid hormones like insulin and serotonin are water soluble and cannot enter the cell – instead they act at the surface of the membrane.

Some cancers are hormone related. These include many – although not all – breast cancers, as well as ovarian cancer, cancer of the womb, prostate and testicular cancer. We will look at oestrogen as an example. Work by the International Agency for Research on Cancer (IARC) has found that the three major oestrogen hormones – oestradiol (the main form of oestrogen), oestrone and oestroil – increased the incidence of a range of cancers in animals, particularly mammary tumours. A recent study by researchers at Harvard Medical School and a leading Boston hospital in the USA[31] found high levels of oestradiol together with another two hormones (testosterone and dehydroepiandrosterone) in women who later go on to develop breast cancer. There is evidence linking oestrogens, taken as HRT, to endometrial cancer[32] and the IARC also found a possible increased risk of developing breast cancer following oestrogen therapy.[33] As a result, steroid oestrogens are classified as Group 1 carcinogens.

In the future, hormone testing could predict up to 20 years in advance who is most likely to develop breast cancer. That would allow protective measures to be adopted before the cancer has a chance to develop.

Growth factors

Growth factors are chemicals produced by the body that control cell growth. They perform many vital tasks like promoting healing or making cells grow. In our circulation system, growth factors are held by other substances called *binding proteins* which modulate their action and control their effects – including their potential impact on cancer cells. The risk of cancer rises when we have abnormally high levels of unbound growth factors circulating in our blood.[34]

The same hormone and growth-factor molecules are found in other animals, although they may serve different purposes. For example, the hormone prolactin governs lactation in women who have recently given birth, but in frogs it controls metamorphosis (the way a tadpole turns into the adult animal).[35] Plants also have these signalling molecules which are subtly but significantly different from those of humans and other animals.[36] That is important for reasons we will see later in Step 5.

We manufacture growth factors in our own bodies in the same way that we manufacture hormones like oestrogen and testosterone. Like hormones, growth factors also occur in the food we eat – at least, in food that comes from animals. There is increasing evidence that consuming animal foods increases the levels of circulating, unbound insulin-like growth factor (IGF-1) and hormones (Step 5). That might be the reason a diet high in animal proteins is associated with a higher cancer risk. We will explore this further in Food Factor 5 (page 135).

More about growth factors

There are many different growth factors which are strongly implicated in the development and spread of cancer. Here we use IGF-1 and VEGF as examples.

Insulin-like growth factor 1 (IGF-1). As its name suggests, IGF-1 is chemically similar to insulin. It plays an important role in early development and at puberty, when it stimulates the development of secondary sexual characteristics such as breasts in girls, the enlarged larynx in boys and body hair in both sexes.[37] About 98 per cent of the IGF-1 produced by our bodies is always bound to one or other of six binding proteins. Cancer risk is higher when there is a high level of unbound IGF-1 circulating freely in the blood and lower when there is a high concentration of the binding proteins.[38]

Vascular endothelial growth factors (VEGF). The name refers to the vascular endothelial cells which line the inside of blood vessels and VEGF is important for stimulating the growth of new blood vessels (angiogenesis),[39] making tissue more permeable, enabling the movement of infection-fighting white blood cells called lymphocytes and driving the body's inflammatory response to bacteria and viruses.

Unfortunately, VEGF also promotes the development and spread of cancer. Solid cancers cannot grow beyond 0.5–1 mm without an adequate blood supply. By promoting angiogenesis VEGF ensures that cancer cells have enough oxygen to survive. Increasing permeability makes it easier for cancer cells to squeeze themselves into blood or lymph vessels and spread around the body. High levels of VEGF have been implicated in a poor prognosis in breast cancer.[40]

The latest generations of anti-cancer drugs are designed to block the action of VEGFs, preventing the cancer from growing and metastasising. The first anti-VEGF drug, a monoclonal antibody named bevacizumab (trade name Avastin), was approved in 2004.

Other important growth factors are epidermal growth factor (EGF), nerve growth factor (NGF) and fibroblast growth factor (FGF).

In the following chapters we are going to tell you how to prevent cancer genes switching on and, if they already have, how to turn them down or, better still, switch them off. Throughout the book we shall use the idea of 'seed and soil' – as the famous biologist Louis Pasteur is claimed to have said on his deathbed 'The seed is nothing; the terrain is everything'. In other words, the condition of your body, the terrain or soil, is crucially important in how illness affects you. Simply, if cancer 'seeds' do not have the right soil in which to grow and cause disease, they will wither and die.

step 2
find your balance

Cancer is not something you can just cut out of your body like a wart or an infected appendix, and know that it's gone for good. Because cancer cells can grow out of control they can invade other tissues and establish secondary tumours, often because underlying problems with the chemistry and physiology of our bodies has made us vulnerable. Cancer is a chronic disease, which often reflects ongoing problems with our diet and lifestyle and in the longer term this can affect our body's inner balance – known to doctors as 'homeostasis' – and our whole physiology.[1, 2]

Our body, brain and mind work together as one astonishingly clever and effective system. In this Step we will explain how our body's internal balance systems work and how they can be affected not only by our lifestyle choices, but also by our life experiences and mental state.

understanding homeostasis

The human brain is widely regarded as the most complex object in the known universe. You can think of it as an amazingly sophisticated computer – and it's certainly that, but it is so much more. All day every day, it takes in signals from our surroundings – the things we see, hear, touch, smell and feel – and processes and integrates the information so that we are able to adapt and maintain control of ourselves and our lives. Thanks to our brain, our bodies are able to repeatedly adjust to changes in our physical, social and emotional environment in order to maintain the internal equilibrium or balance that is vital for good health. This adaptive response underlies the resilience of all animals, including humans, to the changing environment around them.

Maintaining this inner balance helps to keep us healthy but it can be disrupted by any number of physical, environmental and emotional factors such as poor diet, personal trauma or environmental pollutants. The latest research is showing how important this is – involving as it does gene expression (epigenetics) which was discussed in Step 1. Such factors can determine for example whether cancer genes are switched on or up regulated, or down regulated and even switched off or blocked.[3]

The complex interplay of factors that affect us has been represented in a map of human experiences by Ken Wilber (Figure 2.1, below).

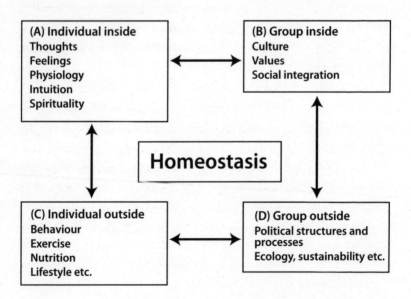

Figure 2.1 Map of human experiences (modified from Wilber, 1996)[4]

Over time, if we don't adapt to changes in our environment and to the physical, social and emotional demands on us, we can end up feeling exhausted and overwhelmed by negative emotions such as fear, frustration, defeat and despair. These feelings can, in turn, disturb our inner balance, leading to physiological changes that affect our body's metabolism.

Metabolism is the total sum of all the biochemical processes that occur within all living organisms – growth, reproduction, and repair – in short everything that's needed to maintain life. There are two possible metabolic end states: anabolic and catabolic (see table overleaf).

In the catabolic state, our bodies break things down, converting complex molecules into smaller units, releasing energy in the process. For example, complex carbohydrates, such as starch, are reduced to sugars like glucose which are essential to provide energy.

In the anabolic state, our bodies build things up and use energy to build large, complex molecules such as proteins from smaller, simpler molecules such as amino acids. In this way, the body is able to create new cells: building up muscle or repairing tissue, for instance.

Anabolism and catabolism are, in essence, the yin and yang of metabolism and are both essential to maintain life. In fact, we tend to be catabolic during the day and anabolic during the night, although as we age, this day/night cycle becomes less pronounced. Maintaining a balance between anabolic and catabolic metabolism is essential to our well-being, as it affects the body's acid/alkali balance, hormone activity and many other metabolic processes. If we get stuck in one state or the other, then all sorts of problems can develop.

Catabolic and anabolic metabolism

Catabolic metabolism in balance	Anabolic metabolism in balance
The body breaks down complex molecules from the food we eat to release energy and provide the building blocks needed to maintain and repair cells.	The body uses the energy released by catabolic metabolism to build new cells and repair damaged tissue: for example, healing wounds.
Releases energy from stored glycogen if needed.	Uses simple molecules such as amino acids to create complex molecules such as proteins.
In starvation, releases energy from stored fat. In extreme starvation will even break down body tissues such as muscle to release energy.	In growing children, provides the new cells needed for building muscle, bone and other tissues.
Gives you plenty of energy during the day.	Enables you to sleep well during the night and awake feeling restored and rested.
Hormones help make sure we can respond swiftly to danger – the 'fight or flight' reaction.	Hormones help maintain the immune system, cardiac health and regulate the level of glucose in the blood.
When the balance gets upset	
If the catabolic metabolism is over-dominant	If the anabolic metabolism is over-dominant
You can become prone to 'burn-out', migraine headaches, insomnia and anxiety.	You may feel tired all the time, become prone to depression, need to urinate frequently especially at night.
You become more prone to infection. Diarrhoea, auto-immune diseases and rheumatoid arthritis are more likely.	You are more likely to develop constipation, high blood pressure and osteoarthritis.

The impact of stress

If we are subjected to stress over a long period of time, our body tends to move to a catabolic state. Catabolic hormones are produced, including cortisol, the 'stress hormone', and adrenalin, the 'fight or flight' hormone. Cortisol increases blood pressure and blood sugar and reduces immune responses, while adrenalin increases the heart rate and strengthens the force of its contractions.

In the catabolic state, the carbohydrates, fats and proteins that make up our bodies are broken down to release energy. This is accompanied by the production of toxic wastes such as lactic acid, carbon dioxide and ammonia under the control of stress hormones such as cortisol and adrenaline. At the same time, our immune system is compromised as the numbers of white blood cells fall and the thymus gland decreases in volume. So homeostasis – keeping our metabolism in balance – is absolutely essential to good health.

the brain-mind-body system

Mission control

Homeostasis is maintained through the brain-mind-body system, a highly organised network of nerves and a range of chemicals. The brain includes its physical structure, cells and chemicals, while the mind includes thoughts, ideas, images and feelings. You might remember from school biology lessons that the brain is connected to the rest of the body through the spinal cord and a collection of nerves known as the peripheral nervous system (PNS). This is designed to relay information from the brain and spinal cord to the rest of the body and back again which, among other things, conveys signals to the body, causing it to move.

In order to understand how homeostasis is maintained or destroyed we need to learn a little more about the human brain.

As well as being physically connected to the rest of the body by nerves, the brain also controls the body chemically using three integrated systems, the nervous (neurotransmitters), endocrine (hormone) and immune (cytokines) systems. The brain is directly connected through the hypothalamus (H) to the master gland of the hormone system, the pituitary gland (P). This means that it can send powerful messages, including surges of adrenaline from the adrenal glands (A), for example, to equip the body for fight or flight in response to sudden threats. If this system, known as the HPA axis, remains switched on for too long so that, for example, adrenaline is released too frequently, our immunity and our health can be undermined because homeostasis has been lost.

In order to understand how homeostasis is maintained or destroyed we need to learn a little more about the human brain and how it works.

the human brain

The logical brain (the cerebrum) is the rational, analytical brain, the part that makes us human. It deals with visual processing, sound and speech, aspects of memory, orientation, calculation and pattern recognition. It integrates functions such as thinking, analysis, conceptualising and planning and enabled humans to develop language as a basis for intellectual tasks such as reading and writing and to understand mathematical concepts.

Feelings are generated in our emotional and instinctive brains (see below), but it is the cerebrum that articulates them and tries to understand and explain them. It can also help us to gain control over our older, more unruly brains through a particularly advanced part of the cerebrum, the prefrontal cortex. This is situated in the frontal lobes (Figure 2.2, opposite) and has many connections with the older brains: the limbic system and the brainstem.

One of the main functions of the prefrontal cortex is the control of our emotions such as anger, panic and rage. However, it can be disabled by sudden threats or long-term strain. Brain-imaging studies carried out over the last few decades have shown that the volume of the prefrontal cortex and its connections with other regions of the brain are reduced when people are subjected to long-term or recurring stress or deprivation – although in many cases these connections can be regenerated.

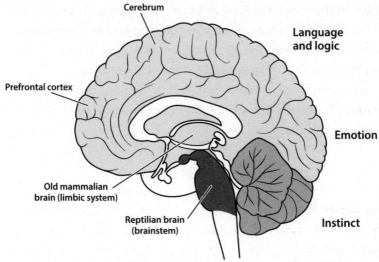

Figure 2.2 *The human brain.*

The emotional brain (the limbic system) is concerned with appetites and urges, pleasant and unpleasant feelings, playful behaviour and emotions for nurturing and protecting the young. It contains the hypothalamus, which triggers the HPA axis and the physical expression of emotions – we can, for example, go hot and cold in response to a sudden emotional shock. The hippocampus, which helps us to remember day-to-day events and find our way around, is also in the limbic system, as is the amygdala, responsible for the formation of powerful stored emotional memories that we cannot recall, which is also known as the brain's fear centre.

The limbic system has a much simpler structure than the cerebrum and processes information much faster, so we can react rapidly to danger. The distinguished neuroscientist, Dr David Servan-Schreiber, illustrated the different roles of the limbic system and cerebrum with the example of how we would react to a piece of wood that resembled a snake: the older brain sets off a fear reaction based on partial or erroneous information before the cerebrum has even begun to determine that the object is harmless.[4]

The brain stem – or reptilian brain – is the oldest, most primitive part of our brain, and developed during the dinosaur era about 300 million years ago. It is concerned with our basic survival and instinctive behaviour such as in aggression, dominance, territoriality, and ritual displays.[5] It controls the autonomic nervous system (ANS) which is outside our conscious control and is responsible for regulating our basic life functions such as blood flow, breathing and heartbeat (see Figure 2.3, below). Over the long term, problems which seriously affect our ANS can destroy our inner balance and undermine our health.

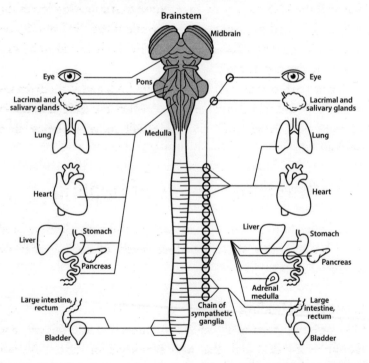

Figure 2.3 *the autonomic nervous system, showing the different 'wiring' of the body when the parasympathetic nervous system is in control (left side of the diagram) and when the sympathetic nervous system is dominant (right side). The two nervous systems are repeated on both sides of the body but are represented in this way on the diagram for clarity.*

The ANS is further divided into the sympathetic nervous system (SNS), which controls fight or flight responses and the parasympathetic nervous system (PNS) which helps maintain normal body functions (Figure 2.3). These two systems work in concert with each other and need to be in balance. For instance, the SNS controls pupil dilation in the eye, whereas the PNS controls pupil contraction. The SNS will decrease urine secretion from the kidney, but the PNS increases it. The SNS increases heart rate and force while the PNS decreases these.

The ANS has two extreme modes of controlling the body. Hence, if the SNS dominates in response to stimulating forces the body is equipped for 'fight or flight' while if the PNS dominates in response to tranquillising influences the body is said to be in a state of 'rest and digest'.

When homeostasis is maintained, the SNS and PNS divisions of the ANS are in balance. However, when the SNS dominates for long periods of time, the body will move to being in a catabolic state.

the three levels of healing

If we are to beat cancer and stay well in the long term we need to understand that there are three levels of healing that we need to address.

Level One Healing

Conventional treatment such as surgery, radiotherapy and chemotherapy deal with the overt symptoms of cancer. We will talk more about these treatments in Step 3.

Level Two Healing

Addressing lifestyle factors such as diet and exercise, which we will cover in Steps 5 to 7.

Level Three Healing

Using talking therapies and mind-body treatments, e.g. acupuncture, yoga and meditation, to help reduce stress and address underlying social, emotional or spiritual problems in our lives. We will cover this in Step 8.

Understanding the three levels of healing

In order to beat cancer we need to integrate conventional medical treatment and other methods of healing to restore our inner balance. Many complementary therapies are aimed at re-establishing homeostasis as a means of helping the body to heal. For example, in Traditional Chinese Medicine patients are treated to rebalance Yang (an aspect of which can be seen as the catabolic use of energy by the SNS) and Yin (which includes the anabolic or building effects of the PNS). This concept of balancing the energy-using SNS and restorative PNS is also fundamental to other traditional forms of healing such as meditation, yoga and Ayurveda.

The success of mind-body treatment for cancer was powerfully demonstrated by research published in 2008 by Professor Dean Ornish, Director of the Preventive Medicine Research Institute in Sausalito, California and Clinical Professor of Medicine at the University of California, San Francisco. This study, on patients with early prostate cancer, demonstrated that 453 genes linked to cancer (oncogenes) were turned off and more than 48 protective genes were turned on when patients were supported by a programme of nutrition, exercise and stress management. Indeed, the importance of dietary and lifestyle factors in promoting or suppressing gene expression (epigenetics) is now being recognised in understanding gene/environmental interactions in several types of cancer, including colorectal, breast, cervical and head and neck cancer.[6]

In the following chapters we will outline the steps you need to take to help prevent and treat cancer using conventional medicine and complementary therapies and by introducing dietary and lifestyle improvements which are all designed to help you improve your resilience and maintain your inner balance.

step 3
choose the right conventional therapies for you

Ultimately, the best cure for cancer is prevention, which is why this book emphasises the role that diet and lifestyle can play in preventing, suppressing or at least delaying the onset of cancer. Cancer is a global problem and more than one in three of us will be diagnosed with cancer at some point in our lives.[1] If you or a loved one fall into this group it is important to understand how your doctors and the rest of the clinical team will manage your diagnosis and treatment. This chapter explains the procedures that you might undergo during investigations for cancer and the treatments you are likely to be offered if the cancer is confirmed.

We want to emphasise that cancer diagnosis and treatment should always be carried out by medically qualified professionals and involve a specialist multi-disciplinary team including an oncologist, surgeon, radiotherapist, pathologist and, sometimes, an endocrinologist who can identify the full extent of the problem and devise an appropriate treatment plan.

worried about symptoms?

If you are worried about any symptoms that could mean cancer, see your GP as soon as possible. Early diagnosis can make all the difference. Cancer survival rates are lower in the UK than in

Europe overall, possibly because people are diagnosed later which then means there may be fewer options for effective treatment.[2] According to the official estimates, over 1,000 lives every year would be saved if Britain matched the European figures.[3]

Act quickly

The chances are that even if you have symptoms, you will not have cancer. For example, only one in 10 people referred for tests for suspected bowel cancer turn out to have the disease. Even so, do not just hope that you will be one of the lucky ones. All sorts of things hold people back from checking out worrying symptoms – embarrassment, concerns about bothering the doctor unnecessarily and sometimes even the fear of bad news. Older people, in particular, can be reluctant to bother their doctor and put symptoms down to 'old age'. However hard it feels, try to put your embarrassment and worries to one side. Your doctor has seen it all before and will not think you are wasting their time if you have symptoms you are concerned about. Remember, the earlier you act, the more likely you are to have a good outcome if you do have cancer. Simply, it is always better to be safe than sorry!

Know the danger signs

All the symptoms listed below can be a sign of cancer so you should always check them out with your GP, especially if they persist for longer than a few weeks.[5] However, remember that they are far more likely to be a symptom of something much less serious – a change in bowel habits, for example, is often caused by a change in diet or an infection.

- An unusual lump or swelling anywhere on your body
- A change in the size, shape or colour of a mole
- A sore that will not heal after several weeks
- A mouth or tongue ulcer that lasts longer than three weeks
- A cough or croaky voice that lasts longer than three weeks

- Persistent difficulty swallowing or indigestion
- Problems passing urine
- Blood in your urine
- Blood in your bowel motions
- A change to more frequent bowel motions that lasts longer than four to six weeks
- Unexplained weight loss or heavy night sweats
- An unexplained pain or ache, including headache, that lasts longer than four weeks
- Breathlessness
- Coughing up blood

In addition, for women:

- An unusual breast change
- Bleeding from the vagina after the menopause or between periods
- Persistent bloating

If your GP is reluctant to refer you for tests and you are still concerned, politely but firmly insist. You know your body and what is normal for you. Most patients are referred after one or two consultations but for some, particularly older people, it may take much longer. In fact almost a third of cancers in the over-70s are diagnosed only after an emergency admission to hospital.[6] Also, a recent study by the UK National Cancer Intelligence Network (NCIN) found that some GPs are three times more likely to refer than others.[7] Some differences are inevitable as some areas have higher cancer rates, and patient groups may be younger. Nevertheless, GP attitudes can differ and experts say that a three-fold variation is worrying. You can check your own GP's referral rates on the NCIN website: http://www.ncin.org.uk/cancer_information_tools/profiles/gp_profiles.aspx

the role of screening

The key to cancer survival is early detection – this is where screening comes in. Although screening rarely provides a definite diagnosis it can detect warning signs before symptoms appear and flag up the need for further investigations.

Screening is not available for all cancers because devising reliable tests is not easy. They have to be designed to ensure the fewest possible false results.

A *false positive result* suggests that cancer is present when it isn't – another reason why further investigations are important.

A *false negative result* can suggest that there is no cancer and all is well when it is not. Screening can miss a cancer if it is too small. So, if symptoms persist go back to your doctor.

The most common screening programmes available in the UK, most of Europe and the USA are for breast, cervical and bowel cancer.

Breast-cancer screening

The NHS currently provides three-yearly breast-cancer screening for women aged 50–70 and by 2016 this will be extended to all women aged 47–73. The screening involves a mammogram – an X-ray of each breast – which can detect changes in breast tissue that may indicate cancers that are too small to be felt either by a doctor or the woman herself.

There has been some controversy over breast-cancer screening, largely because of concerns that over-diagnosis can lead to some women receiving unnecessary treatment.[8] An independent review published in October 2012 found that for every life saved, three women had treatment for a cancer that would never have become life threatening.[9] This matters, because cancer treatments such as surgery, chemotherapy, radiotherapy and hormone therapy can have significant, and sometimes undesirable long-term side effects. On the other hand, there is currently no definitive way of knowing which cancers detected at this early stage will become deadly. Cancer Research UK, which commissioned the review jointly with the Department of Health, says that 'on balance' women should still opt for screening. The review found that more than 1,300 lives are saved every year by breast-cancer screening.[10] Nevertheless, in future, women invited for breast-cancer screening will be given more information about the risks of over-diagnosis so they can make an informed decision.

Bowel-cancer screening

Bowel cancer is cancer of the large bowel, rectum and/or appendix which affects one in 20 people at some time in their lives, and causes around 16,000 deaths every year.[11]

Everyone in their 60s in the UK is now offered a Faecal Occult Blood Test (FOBT) every two years. The test kit, which looks for hidden traces of blood in stools, is sent to your home. It includes paper strips designed to take small smears of stool and you then return these in a secure, hygienic pre-paid envelope to a specialist NHS laboratory for testing. If you have a positive result, you will be invited for further diagnostic tests, often a colonoscopy. FOBT screening reduces the risk of dying from bowel cancer by an estimated 16 per cent.[12]

Cervical-cancer screening

Cervical-smear testing is one of cancer screening's great success stories. Since the screening was introduced in the 1980s, the cases of cervical cancer have decreased steadily.[13] Screening is offered to all women aged 25–64 – those aged 25–49 are invited three-yearly and older women every five years.

The test involves taking a sample of cells from the cervix with a small brush and then testing them for abnormalities. About one in 20 women screened have some changes, although most are not cancer. If changes are detected you will be invited for further investigation. By detecting and treating abnormal 'pre-cancerous' cells, screening can help prevent cervical cancer from developing. Currently around 3,000 women are diagnosed with cervical cancer annually, the majority aged between 30–39. The numbers fall steadily after the age of 40 but increase again slightly after reaching 70.[14]

Prostate cancer – an ongoing debate about screening

The prostate is a walnut-sized gland that produces fluid that carries sperm. Because of its position surrounding the urethra, problems affecting the prostate can also affect urination and sometimes sexual function. Prostate cancer is now the most commonly diagnosed cancer in men and around one in 10 men will develop it in their lifetime. The average age at diagnosis is 70–74.[15] Those with a family history of prostate cancer are more at risk, and so are black-African and black-Caribbean men.[16]

Most experts agree that mass screening for prostate cancer is not a good idea.[17] This is partly because the available test is not reliable enough and the risk of over-diagnosis could mean that some men could face unnecessary treatment with drastic life-changing consequences. However, several countries, including the UK, offer an *informed choice programme*. If you are worried about prostate cancer or have a family history of the disease, you can ask your GP for a Prostate Specific Antigen (PSA) test. This is a blood test which measures the levels of PSA, a protein in the blood which is produced by normal prostate cells but which may occur at high levels if cancer is present (although it can also be raised by infection or after exercise or sexual activity).

Your GP will talk you through the pros and cons of PSA testing as the value of the test is still hotly debated. There is a high risk of false alarms. PSA can be produced in the body by other organs and under conditions that may not be cancer.[18] Also, cancer can be missed (up to one in five men with prostate cancer have normal PSA levels). If the results are positive or uncertain you may have a repeat test and, if cancer is suspected, be asked to attend for further investigations. Some prostate cancers, especially those in the 70+ age group, are slow growing and may be safely left untreated providing they are carefully monitored, known as 'watchful waiting'.[19]

getting a cancer diagnosis

Diagnosing cancer is a multi-step process. The aim is not just to determine whether or not you have cancer but, if you do, what type of cancer, how aggressive it is, whether it has spread (metastasised) and if so where from and where to. Diagnostic tests will help your medical team determine the most appropriate treatment, how best to plan it and how to monitor its effectiveness.

There are three main diagnostic methods:

- **Imaging** – taking pictures to determine the affected organs
- **Biopsy** – taking small tissue samples so that the cancer cells can be examined, commonly under a microscope
- **Body fluids and excrement** – a small amount of fluid (most commonly, blood and urine) and stool tests can be used to check for abnormal cells and tumour markers

The tests that are used, and the order in which they are given, depend on the type and stage of the cancer.

Imaging
Imaging techniques, methods of producing pictures of the body, are used both to detect cancers and to help determine its extent.

- X-rays are often used in the early detection of cancer – mammograms, for example, use X-rays to look for abnormalities in the breast.
- Computed tomography (CT) scans can give a more accurate picture of the body. By taking lots of pictures from different

angles CT scanning generates a three-dimensional picture that can show where the tumour is, and how large it is. Sometimes, with brain or lung tumours for example, the patient will be injected with a dye or mildly radioactive substance so that detail shows up better. CT scans use more ionising radiation than regular X-rays so there is a risk, albeit a low one, that repeated CT scans might eventually cause a second cancer.[20] You should therefore try to avoid repeated CT scans, especially if you have previously shown any sensitivity to such radiation (see Step 7).

- Ultrasound imaging uses high-frequency sound waves which reflect differently off different tissues in the body. The reflected waves are converted into a visual image of the part of the body scanned. Ultrasound imaging is most effective in detecting tumours in the abdomen, breast, liver and kidneys.[21]

- Magnetic resonance imaging (MRI) scanners look like a narrow tunnel that you go into head or feet first, depending on the area being scanned. MRI uses a large rotating magnet and special detector to produce high-resolution images of soft tissue such as ligaments, tendons and nerves as well as of brain, bone and breast tumours. An intravenous injection may be used to enhance the image. Unlike CT or X-ray, MRI is non-ionising.[22]. People suffering from claustrophobia can find MRI difficult and more patient-friendly 'open' MRI machines are now available in some hospitals.

- Positron emission tomography (PET) creates computerised images of the state of metabolism in tissues. Before a PET scan you will have an injection of radioactive labelled sugar.[23] Cancer cells use a lot more sugar than normal cells so the cancer cells take up the radioactive sugar preferentially. The scanner can then create three-dimensional biochemical images of the body including tumours. PET can detect tiny functional changes before anatomical changes can be seen with either CT or MRI scans, and is often used in combination with these techniques.[24] The main advantage of PET is that the tissues that it shows up are more likely to be cancerous whereas the other scans cannot readily distinguish between cancer and other anatomical abnormalities, such as scar tissue. Although PET also involves ionising radiation, this is at a lower level. Nevertheless, it is best to avoid too many scans.[25]

Biopsy

A biopsy involves taking small pieces of tissue from almost any part of the body where cancer is suspected and examining it under the microscope to look for cancer cells and also to identify any genes or proteins that may be indicative of the cancer's growth. This information will help to determine the best course of treatment. A sample of normal tissue may also be taken for comparison. Repeat biopsies may be necessary to monitor the effectiveness of the therapy and to make changes if necessary.

Body fluids and excrement

A variety of body fluids such as blood, lung, peritoneal and excrement (urine and stool) can be used to detect cancer. For example, as well as being used to diagnose leukaemia and other blood cancers, blood tests can detect, directly or indirectly, cancer cells that have escaped from the primary tumour.[26]

Full blood count (FBC)

This measures the number of red cells, white cells and platelets in your blood.[27] Red cells carry oxygen, white cells fight infection, and platelets help the blood to clot in order to stop bleeding. A FBC is done to check general health, for the early diagnosis of cancers such as leukaemia and lymphoma, and to check for treatment side effects. For example, chemotherapy might alter the white-cell count.[28]

Liver-function test (LFT)

The liver performs essential tasks including storing nutrients, converting fat to energy, producing bile and other useful chemicals,

Towards better diagnosis and treatment

Techniques of cancer diagnosis are constantly being improved, with imaging becoming more accurate, biopsies less invasive, and new tumour markers identified. Completely new diagnostic techniques are being developed – here are just a few of those that show great promise for the future.

- *Circulating tumour cells (CTCs).* Cancer cells that travel in the blood stream can now be isolated from just a few millilitres of blood and counted to help measure the progression of the disease and the effectiveness of treatment.[31]

- *DNA microarrays.* It is now possible to screen our 22,000 genes simultaneously on a single computer chip, smaller than the size of a stamp.[32] The technique provides useful information about the epigenetic[33] changes in gene expression triggered by external environmental factors, the presence of mutations or an altered gene pattern – all of which can indicate cancer. The information can also be used to determine which treatment is most likely to be effective – another step towards personalised medicine.

- *microRNAs.* These are small strands of genetic material that control the conversion of genes to proteins, rather than make proteins themselves.[34] There may be over 1,000 miRNAs controlling around 60 per cent of our genes. They can be detected in blood or tissue and changes in their patterns of expression can indicate the presence of cancer.[35] Finding new ways to manipulate miRNAs – for example to block or switch off cancer genes – may also provide exciting new ways to treat cancer.

- *Metabonomics.* This method measures subtle changes in body fluids that accompany all the chemical reactions in the body.[36] Since some of these changes can occur even before it is possible to detect a tumour, it could help in the early detection of cancer.[37]

making blood proteins, helping blood to clot and breaking down harmful substances. Blood tests can reveal problems with any of these processes that may be caused by the indirect effects of cancer.[29] A LFT may be performed to check general health in cancer patients or whether cancer may be present in the liver.

Tumour markers

Tumour markers are substances, usually proteins, that are produced by a cancer or by the body in response to cancer. The test may show a protein in blood that is normally found in a particular tissue or organ. This may suggest that cancer cells from that tissue or organ are circulating in the blood and the cancer has started spreading. Some tumour markers are produced only by a specific type of cancer, while others may be made by several cancer types.[30]

Genetic tests

People with a family history of breast, ovarian or bowel cancer may be offered a blood test to see if they carry the gene associated with that type of cancer. This is called 'predictive testing' because it can be carried out before cancer develops. It is usually possible in the UK on the National Health Service only if you have a living relative who has been diagnosed with cancer and is willing to be tested first.[38]

Urine tests

These check for the presence of blood, various proteins and other substances in urine. The presence of blood may be caused by an infection, but it may be a sign of a urological tumour such as cancer of the bladder, kidney or prostate.[39] Some of these cancers can be fast-growing, so following up the presence of blood in urine can save a life.

Analysis of electrolytes, such as the ratio of sodium to potassium in the blood, can also be indicative of the body's biochemical balance.[40]

Other body fluids such as lymph and the fluid from the lung or abdominal cavities may be analysed for abnormal cells or tumour markers, depending on the type of cancer suspected.[41]

cancer treatment

Every cancer is different – and so is every patient. The molecular profile of cancers can vary enormously and, similarly, individual patients may respond differently to the same treatments. That is why the emphasis today is increasingly on personalised medicine. Your medical team will use the information they have gathered from the various diagnostic tests, together with your medical history and their own knowledge and expertise, to decide on the best treatment for you. There may be more than one option – you may be invited to take part in a clinical trial of a new treatment for example – but you should always be fully involved in deciding the treatment plan. The final decision about treatment will be yours.

Cancer treatment is like waging a war in which the enemy, because of its stem-cell characteristics, is capable of transforming itself in the middle of a battle. The more detail oncologists have about the cancer, particularly its molecular characteristics, the better armed they are to attack it in a way that is the most effective. This means not just deciding on the best treatments – but the order in which to give those treatments. Such a strategy needs considerable experience and the most up to date knowledge and training, which is why specialist cancer centres, ideally staffed with research-active doctors, are so important.

Surgery
Whether or not you have surgery will depend on the type of cancer you have, where the tumour is and how far it has spread. If the cancer is 'localised', confined to one area – an early-stage melanoma or a small breast lump for example – surgery to remove the tumour may be the only treatment that is needed. In general,

the earlier the cancer is found, the easier it is to remove. But the extent of the surgery will depend not just on the size of the tumour, but also on its grade – in other words how abnormal the cells look under the microscope and how likely they are to spread. The tumour grade is one of the key characteristics that your team will assess during the diagnostic process.[42] A high-grade cancer, which is likely to spread quickly and aggressively, is likely to be treated with more extensive surgery than a low-grade one. In the case of breast cancer, for example, that might involve *mastectomy*, removal of the whole breast.[43] Whether local or radical surgery is carried out, it is important that the surgery removes the tumour with a clear margin – a cancer-free area around the tumour – usually about 2 cm wide. This is confirmed by the pathologist after surgery. In a new development, cancer cells can be labelled and then identified using special spectacles to facilitate the surgical removal of the tumour.[44]

If the cancer has already spread, surgery may no longer be an option as simply cutting out the tumour will not be enough. This is the case in high-grade non-Hodgkin's lymphoma and small-cell lung cancer, which usually spread quickly. Again, this emphasises the need for early detection and expert opinion in deciding whether to operate or not.

Sometimes your doctors will suggest treating the cancer before surgery to make it shrink. This might be done with chemotherapy or, in the case of hormone-dependent cancers, with hormone therapy. The treatment might need to continue after surgery to reduce the chance of the disease returning. Cancer cells may escape from the tumour during surgery and remain in the body; this is sometimes called 'minimal residual disease'.[45] If this happens, these remaining cells may eventually re-grow into another tumour. Around a quarter of breast cancer cases re-occur even after radical surgery.[46] This is what happened in Jane's case. So, it is important to remain vigilant, even after the cancer goes into remission (see Step 10).

Surgery is far more sophisticated than it was even 20 years ago – as well as a blade or scalpel, your surgeon has an array of other tools.

Laser surgery is often used for cancers of cervix, larynx, liver, lung, rectum and skin. It reduces bleeding and speeds up healing, since it seals the blood vessels. Another alternative is **cryosurgery** which involves the use of liquid nitrogen to freeze and destroy the tumour[47] making it relatively easy to remove.

Electrosurgery uses pulses of high-frequency electrical current to destroy cancer cells.[48] Easy access to the tumour is important, so this technique is most commonly used for skin and mouth cancers. Like laser surgery and cryosurgery, electrosurgery causes minimal bleeding, and can be repeated if necessary.

Mohs surgery, named after the American surgeon who introduced it,[49] is a microscopically controlled procedure in which skin containing the cancer is removed layer by layer. As each layer is removed, the surgeon checks it under a microscope. When no more abnormal cells can be seen, the surgery can be stopped. It is particularly useful in a situation when as much healthy tissue needs to be spared as possible, for example around the eye. Its success rate is very high.

In laparoscopic or keyhole surgery, the surgeon makes a tiny cut and uses a microscope to locate the tumour which is then removed either by cutting or using a laser.[50] A variation called *thorascopic surgery* might be used in the chest, for example if a lung has collapsed due to fluid build-up. Fluid can be drained, and small tumours on the surface of the lung removed. For early-stage lung cancer, this has proved to be effective and minimally invasive.

Other types of surgery used in cancer treatment include *cosmetic surgery*, because operations for cancer can sometimes cause disfigurement, particularly mastectomy and surgery affecting the face.[51] *Reconstructive surgery* is used to improve function, cosmetic appearance and thus quality of life.[52] In cases of advanced cancer, *palliative surgery* may be carried out to reduce symptoms and improve quality of life and, in some cases, extend life.

Chemotherapy

Chemotherapy simply means drug treatment ('chemo' refers to one or more chemical molecules; 'therapy' means treatment). There are more than 50 types of chemotherapy medication, which work in one of two ways – they either inhibit cancer cells from dividing and reproducing, or they 'trick' the cell into self-destruction.[53]

Chemotherapy might be the main treatment for a particular cancer, but it is often used in combination with other drugs or with radiotherapy. Different treatments use different processes to destroy cancer cells and, together, they may stand a better chance of working than just one on its own. There is less chance of the cancer developing resistance if two or more drugs are given at the same time.[54]

Chemotherapy can be used before surgery to shrink the cancer (which also helps to ensure that it responds to the particular drugs used) as well as after surgery or radiotherapy to destroy any remaining cancer cells. For patients with advanced cancer, chemotherapy might be used to relieve the symptoms and slow disease progression.

Planning your chemo

Chemotherapy is different from medicines such as antibiotics or pain killers which are pre-prepared, with thousands of people taking the same medicine in more or less the same dose every day. Because every cancer patient is different and every cancer is different, each person will have their own unique chemotherapy prescription. Although we can give you general information about chemotherapy here, your doctor or cancer nurse is the person to answer any questions and concerns you have about your treatment.

Your chemotherapy regime and dosage are calculated by measuring your height and weight, and taking blood tests to check your general health and the levels of any cancer markers.

Chemotherapy drugs can affect your bone marrow, where blood cells are manufactured, so your levels of red and white blood cells and platelets might be checked. Depending on the type of cancer you have and the particular drugs being used, there might be other blood tests too.

Most chemotherapy is given either as tablets or intravenously – where the drug is delivered directly into the blood stream using a thin flexible tube called a *canula* which is inserted into a vein but removed after treatment. More rarely it is injected directly into a specific organ such as the bladder[55] or administered as a cream for skin cancer.[56]

Your oncologist will also plan the number of treatment cycles you will need over a certain period of time.[57] If this involves intravenous chemotherapy, you will probably have regular sessions over a period of a few weeks, with a break of two to three weeks in between. If you are taking tablets or capsules, you might take a smaller dose daily for several weeks or months before having a rest period.

The reason for planning treatment in cycles is because chemotherapy drugs are very powerful and, as well as destroying cancer cells, they can also attack other fast-growing cells (see section on *Side Effects*, page 71).[58] The breaks between treatments give tissues time to recover. Repeated doses are needed to progressively decrease the size of the tumour.

It is important that you tell your oncologist or chemo nurse before treatment if you are taking (or plan to take) any other medication, including anything you buy over the counter such as vitamins or supplements, herbal or alternative remedies or even common medicines like aspirin (see Step 4). Any of these might react with your chemotherapy drugs.[59]

Chemo sessions
Do not feel you are being silly or cowardly if the thought of chemotherapy frightens you. Everyone is scared, especially before

the first session. If you can, take a family member or friend with you; it can make all the difference, especially when you have to wait around for test results. You might also need someone to drive you to and from the hospital. Most people are able to drive themselves home after chemotherapy but for your first appointment it is better to be safe than worry about feeling unwell or shaky and so unable to get home.

Before every chemo session you will be given a blood test to check your levels of red and white blood cells and platelets, and your kidney and liver function will be measured. You will need to have the test results before your chemo, because if anything is not working as well as it should, there is a risk of more side effects. If the test shows that your red-cell count is too low, you might have a blood transfusion and if the white-cell and platelet counts are too low, your treatment may need to be delayed because further chemotherapy could push them down to dangerous levels. In this case, you will probably be asked to come back for another test a week later.

It might be possible to have the blood tests on the day before treatment to cut down on waiting. If you have to travel a long way to a specialist cancer centre, talk to your chemo nurse about the possibility of having the tests done at your local hospital.

Once the doctors know that your blood-cell count is fine, your chemotherapy will be prepared. As each prescription is unique it will not be made up until you are ready for treatment. For most people treatment takes several hours and they can go home afterwards. Some people can have their chemotherapy at home, although this depends on the treatment and the patient and the services available locally. A minority of patients may need to stay in hospital for chemotherapy.

Most patients have a temporary canula inserted into a vein to deliver the chemotherapy but some people are given a *central line* (sometimes called a Hickman line) – a fine canula which is inserted into your chest and connected to one of the veins near the heart. This is left in place for the duration of the treatment; it does not hurt and will not interfere with everyday living. You will be given special plastic plasters to prevent it getting wet when bathing or showering.

In a similar procedure, a *Peripherally Inserted Central Catheter* (PICC) is usually put into your arm.[60] Another alternative is an *implanted port* or *portocath*[61] where a small chamber is inserted under the skin and connected by a thin tube to a nearby vein. Some people prefer this method because nothing is visible and they do not have to worry about taking care of a central line or catheter. Others prefer the catheter method because they do not like needles.

If the chemo needs to be delivered slowly over a long period of time (usually hours) and you are staying in hospital, you will probably have an *infusion pump* attached to the canula.[62] The pump is usually on a drip stand on wheels, so you can walk around with it. There are also small, portable pumps that you can take home. Some patients prefer pumps, because everyday life is not disrupted and there is no need for frequent hospital visits.

Although problems are rare, very occasionally fluid can leak into the surrounding tissue. Tell your nurse straight away if your drip stops running or if the area around a canula gets sore.

Home treatment

If you are having tablets or capsules, you can usually take them at home. You will be told how to take them and store them. It is important to ensure that your drugs are safe from children or pets. If you miss a dose ask your pharmacist what to do. Wash your hands after touching a tablet and always flush the lavatory after using it because chemotherapy drugs are excreted in the urine and stool. If for any reason you cannot take the medicine, or you are sick after taking it, contact your chemo nurse or oncologist immediately.

Monitoring your treatment

The blood tests before every chemo session show how your body is reacting to treatment. At intervals, you will have other blood tests and possibly scans or X-rays to assess how well the treatment is working. If necessary, your oncologist may want to change the drug or look at other options.

Side effects

One of the reasons people feel anxious about chemotherapy is because of side effects. Because these drugs work by targeting fast-dividing cells (a key characteristic of cancer cells) they also affect other fast-growing cells such as hair follicles and the cells lining the gut. That is why people receiving chemotherapy can find their hair falls out and they may feel nauseous. Some people may also experience fatigue. However, not all chemotherapy drugs have these effects, and not all patients experience them. What's more there are now good treatments, such as anti-nausea drugs,[63] that minimise side effects. Most side effects are temporary and clear up after treatment although some may continue, at least for some weeks. Whether or not you have side effects has nothing to do with how well the chemotherapy is working.

New developments in chemotherapy

One of the latest developments in cancer treatment – although not suitable for all cancers – is direct infusion of the chemotherapy drug into the tumour or a blood vessel feeding the tumour.[64] Called *isolated infusion* or *embolisation therapy*, this means that a larger dose can be delivered with a smaller risk of damaging normal tissues. Advanced technologies such as nanoparticles[65] and electrochemotherapy[66] are starting to be used with drugs to increase their effectiveness.

Radiotherapy

Radiotherapy uses radiation to kill cancer cells[67] by damaging their DNA. It can also act indirectly by interacting with water molecules inside cells, creating highly reactive and unstable *free radicals* which further disrupt the cell.[68]

Radiotherapy may be the main treatment, which aims to destroy the cancer, or it can be used to prevent it coming back – after surgery for example. It is often given before, during or after chemotherapy.

Computers are increasingly used to maximise the accuracy of radiotherapy treatment. Multi-dimensional 'stereotactic'[69] and 'conformal'[70] radiotherapy use computers to direct the radiation to precisely where it is needed so as to avoid damaging surrounding healthy tissues.

Radiotherapy treatment works best when cancers are localised and superficial – it may not be suitable for cancers that have already spread because it cannot be applied to the whole body, or even a large part of it, without doing harm. It is most successful with highly radiosensitive cancers such as leukaemia, most lymphomas and some ovarian and testicular cancers (although it is rarely used for the latter). Other types of cancer are only moderately radiosensitive and require significantly higher doses to have an impact.[71]

Success also depends on the size of the tumour. Smaller cancers respond better than larger ones. For this reason, you may be advised to have surgery to remove as much as possible of the cancer before radiotherapy starts. Another approach is to give chemotherapy first to shrink the tumour. Radiosensitising chemotherapy drugs may also be used during a course of radiotherapy.[72]

There are several different types of radiotherapy, and new techniques are being developed continually. Like chemotherapy, radiotherapy involves a series of sessions following the initial consultation. Your doctors are best placed to explain what these are and what options are available. Do not hesitate to ask for more information if you feel confused about what they are telling you.

Like any other treatment, radiotherapy can have adverse side effects depending upon the part of the body being treated. Always tell your doctor or cancer nurse if you think you are experiencing side effects.

High-intensity focused ultrasound (HIFU). Ultrasound is frequently used for diagnosis – ultrasound scans in pregnancy for example. But at much higher frequencies, ultrasound produces heat that can be used to destroy tumour tissue.[73] By using focused beams from several sources operating at different angles, a precise radiation dose can be delivered to a small target area with minimal damage to the surrounding normal tissue. HIFU is non-invasive and can be used for treatment of cancers of head, neck, lung, brain, breast, liver, bone and prostate. It has also been used in palliative care of some cancers (e.g. pancreatic) and secondary bone tumours.[74] HIFU can also be given with hyperthermia-triggered drug delivery – combining chemotherapy with exposing tissue to high temperature to help destroy cancer cells.[75]

Other types of radiation therapy include 'stereotactic radiosurgery', for example the 'gamma knife' (a highly focused array of gamma rays directed onto the tumour)[76] and 'brachytherapy' (implanting short-lived radioactive 'seeds' directly into the tumour).[77] In intensity-modulated radiation therapy (IMRT), sophisticated software and hardware are used to vary the shape and intensity of the radiation so as to treat the diseased area with precision, with minimal damage to surrounding tissues.

Other treatments
Hormone therapy
Some cancers depend on hormones to help them grow – most commonly breast, prostate, testicular, ovarian and uterine cancer. Many breast cancers, for example, are known as hormone receptor positive cancers, as their growth is driven by the hormone oestrogen, while prostate cancer is dependent on the male hormone testosterone to help it grow. Hormone therapy aims to

block the effects of these hormones on cancer cells. This can be achieved either by stopping hormone production by removing the organ that produces it – such as removing the ovaries to prevent the production of oestrogen – or by using drugs.[78] These can be used to suppress its production. For example, aromatase inhibitors block the action of the enzyme aromatase which normally produces oestrogen from androgens.[79] Another example is tamoxifen, which is an oestrogen receptor blocker, stopping oestrogen from locking onto its receptors on breast cancer cells.[80]

While some hormones encourage the growth and survival of tumour cells, there are others that can help to stop cancer growth. *Progestins*, which have a similar structure to progesterone, have been used to treat advanced breast cancer, endometrial cancer and prostate cancer.

Hormone therapy is not a cure-all, as cancers can eventually become hormone resistant.[81] For example, the useful period of tamoxifen is usually around five years, although there has been a recent suggestion for it to be extended. Importantly, therefore, all this type of medication should be adjusted periodically and this requires expert decision making.

Monoclonal antibodies

Sometimes called 'magic bullets', monoclonal antibodies are now some of the most successful cancer drugs (see table opposite). *Monoclonal* simply means that all the antibody molecules are exactly the same. These drugs are engineered to attach themselves to specific proteins on the surface of cancer cells to destroy them. They can disrupt certain biological processes in cancer cells and so stop them growing or kill them. For example, rituximab (trade names Rituxan and MabThera) sticks to CD20, a protein found primarily on the surface of leukaemia and lymphoma cells[82] enabling the cells of the immune system to find and destroy the cancer. Bevacizumab (Avastin) binds to VEGF, a protein that helps cancers to develop blood vessels, so that blocking it suppresses the growth of the tumour.[83] Trastuzumab (Herceptin) is another well-known monoclonal antibody drug, which is useful against some breast and stomach cancers.[84] Although monoclonal antibody drugs are effective, they may damage other tissues so their side effects must be carefully monitored. They also tend to be expensive and oncologists may resist prescribing them. If you feel that you would benefit from treatment with such drugs, you should insist!

FDA–approved monoclonal antibodies for cancer treatment

Source: Food and Drug Administration (FDA),
Center for Drug Evaluation and Research
http://www.fda.gov/AboutFDA/CentersOffices

Name of drug – common name (and trade name)	Type of cancer it treats
Alemtuzumab (Campath)	Chronic lymphocytic leukaemia
Bevacizumab (Avastin)	Cancers of brain, colon, kidney and lung
Cetuximab (Erbitux)	Colon cancer Head and neck cancers
Ibritumomab (Zevalin)	Non-Hodgkin's lymphoma
Ofatumumab (Arzerra)	Chronic lymphocytic leukaemia
Panitumumab (Vectibix)	Colon cancer
Rituximab (Rituxan)	Chronic lymphocytic leukaemia Non-Hodgkin's lymphoma
Tositumomab (Bexxar)	Non-Hodgkin's lymphoma
Trastuzumab (Herceptin)	Breast cancer Stomach cancer

Immunotherapy

Your immune system is your body's most important defence against disease. However, because cancer cells are damaged versions of your own cells the immune system does not recognise or attack them. Immunotherapy drugs boost the immune system or trick it into attacking the cancer. Additionally, special immune cells in the blood can be isolated, harvested in laboratory conditions and then transfused back into the patient, resulting in a stronger immune response.[85]

Some natural products have been shown to stimulate elements of the immune system. The mushroom *Agaricus subrufescens,* for example, contains beta-glucans, which are thought to interact with receptors on immune cells and stimulate the production of natural killer cells and macrophages – white blood cells which 'gobble up' invaders. Spirulina, a blue-green alga, may also boost the immune response and work against cancer.[86]

Vaccination

Scientists have been working hard to develop anti-cancer vaccines. There are now effective vaccines against HPV (the human papillomavirus), the cause of most cervical cancers, and hepatitis B virus, which can cause liver cancer.[87] Prostate cancer that no longer responds to hormone therapy and is difficult to treat responds to a procedure called 'Sipuleucel-T'.[88] This involves taking some of the patient's own white blood cells, mixing them with a protein that encourages them to attack prostate cancer cells and putting them back into the body. Ipilimumab is used for the treatment of melanoma and works by stimulating the body's T cells, which help fight disease.[89]

Tyrosine kinase inhibitors

Tyrosine kinases (TKs) are enzymes which, as we explained in Step 1, help to send signals in cells and play a key role in encouraging cancers to develop. Tyrosine kinase inhibitors (TKIs) block these enzymes and can thus inhibit cancer growth.[90] For example, Imatinib (Gleevac), which can be used to treat a range of cancers including some leukaemias and GIST, a rare type of stomach cancer, works by targeting different TKs, depending on the cancer treated. This prevents the growth of cancer cells and leads to their death by 'apoptosis' – the cells literally self destruct.[91] Similarly, Gefitinib (Iressa) is used against non-small-cell lung cancer by inhibiting a protein called EGF receptor.[92] Erlotinib (Tarceva) is used to treat pancreatic cancer that has spread and non-small-cell lung cancer.[93] Lapatinib (Tykerb) is used for advanced breast cancer and works by inhibiting both EGF receptors and HER2.[94] More TKIs are currently being developed.[95, 96, 97]

Stem-cell and bone-marrow transplants

Hematopoietic stem cell (HSC) transplantation (or bone marrow transplant) is a therapy used to treat multiple myeloma, lymphoma and leukaemia.[98] It involves taking stem cells from the bone marrow, peripheral blood or umbilical cord blood, using high dose chemotherapy to kill the cancer cells in the bone marrow and then transplanting the stem cells back into the body. The transplanted stem cells can then become white or red blood cells or platelets.[99] Such transplants may be the primary treatment (as in multiple myeloma) or may be carried out after other treatments have failed.

During the transplantations, the patient's own immune system is completely suppressed so that the transplant will not be rejected.

There are two important risks associated with stem cell transplants. First, the initial high-dose chemotherapy can leave the patient open to all possible infections or can result in bleeding. Second, following the transplant, the immune-suppressed patient needs extreme protection from outside germs. Deciding on this kind of therapy is a delicate balancing act because sometimes the risk of infection can be greater than the chance of the transplant working.

Supportive therapies

There are a number of therapies used to support the main treatment and/or to counteract its side effects. Biphosphonates are phosphate-rich drugs prescribed to maintain bone strength by reducing the loss of calcium from bone. They may be used to protect and strengthen bones in breast and prostate cancer, both of which can spread to the bones.[100] Some cancer treatments such as anti-oestrogen therapy can weaken bones, and biphosphonates may be prescribed to protect bones.

- **A blood transfusion** may be needed to treat anaemia, a reduction in the number of red blood cells that can affect people with cancer.[101] This can be due to the cancer itself or the treatment used.
- **Erythropoietin treatment** is an alternative to blood transfusion for anaemia which can develop towards the end of chemotherapy.[102] Erythropoietin is a hormone produced naturally in the intestine which stimulates the body to make red blood cells.
- **Plasma exchange** is used for some cancers like myeloma, where patients can develop high levels of abnormal proteins called immunoglobulins.[103] This can make their blood very thick, causing headaches, blurred vision and tiredness.[104] If this happens, the blood plasma, rather than whole blood, is exchanged, to reduce the level of immunoglobulins and relieve symptoms. Plasma exchange may also be used in cases of myeloid leukaemia, where the white-blood-cell count is very high.[105]
- **Platelet transfusions** may be needed to prevent your platelet count from falling too low. Some cancers, especially leukaemia, can cause a decrease in the level of platelets in the blood and this can also be a side effect of chemotherapy. Very low platelet counts can cause nose bleeds, bleeding gums, and heavy periods, for example.
- **Granulocyte colony-stimulating factor (GCSF)** may be used to stimulate bone marrow to make the white blood cells needed to fight infection. This may be needed if significant numbers of white blood cells have been lost during chemotherapy or radiotherapy.[106]

- **Steroid treatment** can help make chemotherapy more effective and suppress adverse (including allergic) reactions to chemotherapeutic drugs.[107] Steroids (or corticosteroids) are hormones naturally produced in the body by the adrenal glands[108] which help reduce inflammation as well as controlling other functions such as balancing salt and fluid levels.

Emerging therapies

New therapies for cancer are emerging all the time but a major focus at the moment is personalised therapy so the treatment is tailored to the particular cancer and to the individual patient and their genetic make-up.[109] The number of potential targets for treatment is also increasing so that the cancer may be treated at any stage of its development (see Step 1).

Gene therapy

Gene therapy broadly aims to do one of two things:

- to repair faulty genes and/or
- to regulate genes that are expressed at abnormal levels (i.e. too much or too little – epigenetics).[110]

In a recent, exciting development, it was found that the drug vemurafenib could stop the action of a faulty gene, *BRAF*, which causes the over-production of a protein, which, in turn, drives growth in advanced melanoma.[111] More experimental remedies are using specific inhibitors to silence over-expressed genes and/ or gene products. New drugs targeting the processes that control the level of gene expression (i.e. epigenetic drugs) are also in development.[112]

Microbial therapies

The idea of using bacteria as a potential cancer therapy dates back to the late 1800s, when doctors noticed that gangrenous patients 'cured themselves' of tumours. There are three types of microbial therapies.

First, micro-organisms like bacteria and viruses can be used to attack cancer cells specifically.[113] Bacteria can be used to attack cancers that are large enough to be dead ('necrotic') in the middle. This is because certain bacteria cannot grow well, or in some cases cannot grow at all, when oxygen is present. Since growing tumours lack oxygen, such bacteria will thrive and grow in cancerous tissue, consuming the tumour in the process.

Second, some chemical substances produced by micro-organisms have anti-cancer properties.[114] Chemicals produced by microbes can convert a harmless 'pro-drug' into an active agent with anti-cancer effects.[115] Because the bacteria can survive only inside the tumour the pro-drugs can be given in large amounts.

Third, harmless viruses can be engineered to deliver anti-cancer genes to tumours.[116] Scientists have developed such viruses to carry drugs to manipulate genes in the tumour.[117] Another approach involves the use of 'oncolytic' viruses to infect and kill cancer cells.[118]

Photodynamic therapy

Photodynamic therapy (PDT) is used to treat some cancers[119] and has the advantage of being minimally invasive and non-toxic. The patient is given a drug containing a photosensitiser which is taken up preferentially by the cancer cells because they are more active than normal cells. When the cancer is subsequently exposed to light of a particular wavelength the chemical photosensitiser produces a type of reactive oxygen species that kills the cancer cells. Photodynamic therapy can be used topically for superficial cancers, like skin cancers. In order to treat deeper tumours, endoscopes (light-bearing tubes) are used because the light used for PDT has limited penetration.[120]

Some photosensitisers have a high affinity for the vascular endothelial cells which line the circulatory system, so PDT can be targeted on to the blood vessels supplying tumours and hence suppress angiogenesis.[121] The FDA has approved the photosensitising agent photofrin for use in treatment of oesophageal and non-small-cell lung cancer.[122] Although PDT is useful, it has its limitations. As it is a 'local' treatment, it cannot be used for cancers that have spread.

Radiofrequency ablation

Radiofrequency ablation (RFA) uses a probe carrying a low-frequency electric current to raise the temperature in the tumour and thus destroy it.[123] RFA is generally used to treat small primary or secondary tumours, eliminating the cancer or reducing its size and relieving symptoms. It has been used to treat tumours of lung,[124] liver,[125] kidney, pancreas,[126] bone[127] and occasionally other organs.[128] RFA may be used as an alternative to surgery if the patient cannot have anaesthetic or if the tumour is near a critical part of the body. It has been combined successfully with locally delivered chemotherapy to treat primary liver cancer. In a modified form, RFA may be used to treat pancreatic cancer.[129]

Electrotherapy

Tumours can also be destroyed by bombarding them with brief pulses of high-voltage electricity, with minimal damage to surrounding tissues.[130] So far, this technique has been applied only to superficial tumours, such as skin cancers (including aggressive melanomas) where the pulses can be delivered easily.[131] Research is underway to see if the technique can be combined with an endoscope to eliminate cancers deeper in the body (especially those that are currently difficult to treat, such as pancreatic cancer).[132]

Nanotechnology

Nanoparticles are extremely small – a nanometre is one millionth of a millimetre – and their minute size means that they can penetrate any part of the body and interact with parts of cells at a fundamental level. This gives them huge potential for cancer treatment. For example, nanoparticles can cross the blood-brain barrier, which many cancer drugs cannot.[133] In one study, iron nanoparticles were coated with a chemotherapy drug and guided, under imaging, into a brain tumour using a magnetic field, enabling the drug to be delivered directly to the tumour while avoiding undesirable side effects.[134] Nanotechnology is now a multi-billion pound industry, and further applications to cancer medicine are predicted.[135]

Neuroactive drugs

In Step 1, we showed that cancer cells are electrically active; and the more aggressive they are the more excitable they are.[136] We know the proteins (and their genes) that generate this electrical hyperactivity. We also know that it is the expression of the voltage-gated sodium channel in its embryonic form that causes cancer cells to start spreading to other parts of the body. Recent findings suggest that blocking these channels in cancer cells can suppress the cancer from spreading.[137] This can be done using simple drugs which are already being used to treat other conditions like epilepsy and cardiac arrhythmia.[138] Even aspirin is proving to be effective in suppressing cancer.[139] It is possible that in a few years we may be able to control cancer spread just by using cheap, non-toxic drugs.[140]

'staying on course' is crucial after treatment ends

In this chapter, we covered the available conventional treatments that a cancer patient may undergo. We also outlined some exciting new developments in cancer treatment. We strongly advise you to follow the advice of your medical team in obtaining the best possible clinical therapy. Following the completion of any regime of therapy, however, it is essential that you take precautions to stay on course. For example, you should follow the dietary and life-style measures discussed in Steps 5 and 6. Step 10 describes how to 'stay on course'. We urge cancer patients to read this carefully and to follow the advice given closely.

This is as far as most conventional medicine available in cancer clinics will take your treatment. In the following sections we shall explain all the additional things that you can do to help yourself, such as modifying your diet and lifestyle. These are increasingly being demonstrated to be powerful factors in healing, and we now understand their importance much better, thanks to the new science of 'epigenetics'.

step 4
know which complementary therapies can help

The term *complementary therapies* covers a wide range of treatments generally not used in conventional Western medicine – everything from acupuncture to visualisation and many others. Although these treatments are popular, generally, however, few of them have been well researched. Consequently, often we do not really know whether or how well a particular 'complementary' therapy works, how it acts on the body or how safe it is.

Surveys have found that around a third of cancer patients use some forms of complementary therapy at some time during their illness to help them deal with the symptoms of cancer and the side effects of treatment. Patients may use them to help combat fatigue, alleviate sleep problems, relieve anxiety, and enable them to cope better psychologically – all areas where complementary therapies intend to prove their worth. However, although some therapies can be beneficial, others are risky – particularly if you are having orthodox treatment at the same time – and a few could be positively dangerous.

What none of them can do, however, is cure cancer. An aggressive cancer is rather like a juggernaut, forging ahead, regardless of the surrounding tissue. You need the power of conventional medicine to stop the juggernaut in its tracks. What the more subtle, often gradual, effects of complementary therapies can do is to ease your progress through treatment, support your recovery afterwards and help to restore your inner balance (Step 2).

For these reasons here is a health warning: Complementary therapies should be just that. They should *complement* your medical care, not *replace* it. For that reason also, we do not like the term 'alternative'! If you come across a practitioner who advises you to give up your conventional treatment, run a mile. Such advice is dangerous. Always tell your medical team if you are planning

Internet research – some guidelines

Many people turn to the internet in their search for effective and additional treatments. There is a huge amount of information relating to complementary cancer treatment and the evidence to support it available on the internet – some of it sound but much of it unreliable and misleading. To help you evaluate any internet-based information, we advise you to ask the following three important questions:

1. How recent is this information? An old remedy that may have been considered okay at the time may no longer be acceptable or may have been shown to be unsafe or ineffective since the information you are reading was published.
2. Was the study or proposal that supports the use of this treatment or remedy published in a reputable journal? Unless an idea has been peer-reviewed effectively there is no sound evidence of its efficacy. We are aware that some scientific ideas, even good ones, can be dismissed by competitors. Nevertheless, if the evidence is there, even the most critical scientist will eventually have to accept it!
3. Has the evidence been replicated elsewhere in other research? Strict scientific discipline requires that the result of a study or experiment cannot be accepted unless it has been replicated independently by others.

to try complementary therapies. There might be unexpected interactions with your conventional care. Even taking vitamins or food supplements can sometimes cause problems.

Be wary of advertising claiming that a therapy or product is 'natural and safe' or '100% safe' and steer well clear of anything that claims it can 'cure' cancer, however many testimonials from grateful patients they produce. The likelihood is that whatever they are selling has not been rigorously tested or researched and that someone is simply keen to get hold of your money. Remember that anything can be posted on the internet. Unlike regular advertising, no one monitors websites to make sure their content is truthful and products are safe. The bottom line is that you should never buy medicines online.

finding complementary therapies on the NHS

Most major National Health Service (NHS) cancer centres in the UK now make at least some complementary therapies available for their patients and sometimes their carers too. Experts have found that many patients cope better – and often recover more quickly – when complementary therapies are used alongside orthodox treatment, together known as *integrated medicine*. Cancer experts appreciate the value of a holistic approach which recognises that cancer patients are not just their illness or the sum of their symptoms, but individuals with varied needs, attitudes to life and views on treatment.

Many NHS doctors positively encourage their patients' use of complementary therapies to support them during treatment and recovery. For example, medical teams at University College London Hospital can refer their patients for aromatherapy, massage, reflexology and reiki, while Royal Marsden Hospital offers acupuncture and art therapy among others. The Christie NHS Foundation Trust in Manchester provides a similar range of therapies, and patients in Birmingham with head and neck cancers have access to a specialist complementary-therapy service. At The Velindre Cancer Centre in Cardiff therapists work alongside healthcare professionals to help people deal with psychological and spiritual concerns that affect their quality of life. They also offer therapies that help alleviate anxiety, pain, side effects and symptoms. Holistic facials and Indian head massage are among the services provided by the Macmillan Cancer Resource Centre linked to the East Cheshire NHS Foundation Trust. These are just a few examples of the complementary therapies provided in hospitals around the country – this list is certainly not exhaustive. If you are interested in using a complementary therapy ask what is available locally. Do not feel embarrassed about discussing it with your medical team even if the therapy you are interested in is not available at your own hospital. Your doctors will only advise against it if they think there is a potential risk involved.

The therapies available on the NHS – and the number of sessions you can have – vary enormously and will depend on where you are being treated. If there is a Macmillan Cancer Centre or Maggie's Centre nearby, you may be able to have complementary therapies free of charge or at a subsidised rate.

how to find a private therapist

If you want to find complementary treatment privately remember that it can be expensive – especially if you are looking for long-term support – and you need to choose very carefully. Finding someone who works, or has worked, in the NHS is a useful indicator of safe, good-quality practice. Ask for an initial consultation before committing yourself, to find out what the therapist is offering, and their experience of working with cancer patients. Check their training and qualifications and that they hold indemnity insurance. There is a voluntary registration system for therapists managed by the **Complementary and Natural Healthcare Council**, which was set up by the government. You can search this register online at cnhc.org.uk

how complementary therapies work

East versus West

Western or orthodox medicine is a system based on experimental science. Treatments are extensively tested before being licensed for routine use. New drugs, for example, are assessed in 'randomised controlled trials' (RCTs) involving double-blind tests in which the new treatment is tested against a placebo (dummy or fake version). Neither the doctor nor the patient knows whether the treatment they are receiving is the real thing or the dummy version to ensure that any 'placebo effect' is eliminated. The placebo effect refers to our bodies' astonishing ability to heal themselves because we expect or believe it will happen.

On the other hand, traditional Eastern medicine, which is the basis of some complementary therapies, is based on thousands of years of observation and hands-on experience and its concepts are dramatically different from the West. Chinese medicine, for example, is based on yin-yang theory, which says that everything is shaped by these two opposing but interdependent and complementary forces. To analyse symptoms a Chinese doctor uses eight principles. These are arranged as four pairs of opposing forces – yin-yang, cold-heat, interior-exterior and excess-deficiency. The Chinese believe that a vital energy called *qi* or *chi* circulates along a system of pathways or meridians and ill-health is caused by blocks or a lack of harmony in this circulation. The traditional Chinese five elements – fire, earth, metal, water and wood – are used to explain how the body works. Each organ in the body is thought to correspond to one of these elements.

In the past none of this has made much sense to Western-trained scientists, yet in China today, traditional medicine is provided alongside – and often integrated with – Western medicine. Eastern and Western scientists are increasingly working together and new treatments have been developed based on ancient Chinese herbal remedies. Indeed it has been suggested that yin and yang represent the physiology of the parasympathetic (yin) and sympathetic (yang) nervous systems and that balancing them helps to restore homeostasis (see Figure 2.3).[1]

Meditation, shiatsu, reflexology and other therapies based on Eastern medicine are now available in some NHS cancer clinics. The integration of Western and Eastern medicine, which has been happening in China for years, is increasingly happening in the West too.

an a to z of complementary therapies

We have grouped together therapies commonly used by cancer patients to relieve symptoms and the side effects of treatment. Some are backed up by good research – but for many there is far less evidence that they are effective. Several alleviate stress, tension and anxiety and may thus help in restoring homeostasis. This is not an exhaustive list but it covers many of the therapies available in NHS hospitals, though no hospital offers all of them.

Acupuncture

Acupuncture is a traditional Chinese treatment, used increasingly in the West and for which there is a growing evidence base.[2] It involves the insertion of very fine needles – about the thickness of a hair – at points along the traditional 'meridians' which may be stimulated by moving them slightly. Although there are about five hundred acupuncture points in the body an acupuncturist will usually use only 10 of these in a typical session which lasts 20 to 40 minutes. Acupuncture has been extensively researched and has been shown to reduce the nausea, fatigue and pain often experienced by cancer patients following surgery and during chemotherapy.[3] The UK National Institute for Clinical Excellence (NICE) now recommends acupuncture as a treatment for chronic lower back pain. It is generally safe, side effects are uncommon and, if they do occur, tend to be minor and transient. An increasing number of physiotherapists are trained in acupuncture and many NHS cancer clinics provide it.

Electro-acupuncture, a modern version of the therapy, involves passing a small electrical current through the acupuncture needle. A RCT on lung- and breast-cancer patients with bone disease found that electro-acupuncture alleviated neuropathic pain, decreased the amount of painkillers needed and improved patients' quality of life.[4] Another study showed that the pain-relieving effect of electro-acupuncture can last months after treatment.[5] Importantly, its action can be observed in brain scans, confirming that the effect is physiological not psychological or due to the placebo effect.[6]

If acupuncture is not available at your local cancer clinic but you would like to try it, make sure you choose a fully trained and experienced acupuncturist. The **British Acupuncture Council** is a reputable body, whose members have completed at least first degree or equivalent level training. Their website provides a searchable register. Visit www.acupuncture.org.uk. Members of the **British Medical Acupuncture Society** are doctors and allied health professionals who practise acupuncture alongside more conventional care. This too has an online register where you can find a local practitioner. Visit www.medical-acupuncture.co.uk.

Traditional Chinese Medicine

Traditional Chinese Medicine (TCM) can be effective, powerful and safe in the hands of well-trained, qualified practitioners – Jane worked in China over a period of 15 years or so and can vouch for that from her personal experience. However, imported Chinese herbal medicines can have serious risks.

We recommend that you do not use herbs or herbal medicines indiscriminately at the same time as having active cancer treatment unless your oncologist agrees. If you are interested in trying TCM at other times, do your homework. Ask the practitioner about their training and if he or she is a member of a recognised body or practitioner association, like **The Association of Traditional Chinese Medicine and Acupuncture (www. atcm.co.uk)** who say that they promote proper professional training and the highest standards of practice. Most importantly, check that they use suppliers who are approved by the Register of Chinese Herbal Medicine, a voluntary scheme that includes an independent audit. At the time of writing, five companies have been approved. However, remember that neither suppliers nor practitioners are subject to statutory regulation like conventional medical practitioners.

Warning – Chinese and other ethnic herbal medicines

There are long-standing and serious concerns about the safety of some imported herbal medicines, particularly those from mainland China, and those promoted on websites which may be based overseas. There is a danger that medicines may be contaminated with toxic heavy metals such as lead, mercury and cadmium or arsenic or toxic herbs – which may look similar to medicinal herbs. In 2010 a woman tragically developed kidney cancer after treating her eczema with a Chinese herbal preparation supplied by a high street Chinese medicine shop.[7] There have been other similar cases in the UK and worldwide – as well as heart attacks, strokes, seizures, kidney and liver damage and, sadly, deaths – caused by poor-quality herbal preparations.[8] We also deplore the use of animal parts for any treatment and believe it will be completely ineffective.

Eating rhino horn has been likened to eating human fingernails, for example.

These issues are not limited to Chinese medicines. Heavy-metal contamination and other toxic substances have been found in Ayurvedic herbal preparations from the Indian sub-continent, and in medicines from Africa.[9]

Herbal preparations may also be adulterated with powerful prescription drugs. Unscrupulous manufacturers do not declare that these are present so the user – and often the practitioner – has no idea what they are taking. One recent US study found aristolochic acid, a primary cause of kidney cancer, in some Chinese herbal medicines.[10] The UK's Medicines and Healthcare Products Regulatory Agency (MHRA), the government body that licenses medicines, has also identified aristolochic acid, as well as steroids, prescription diabetes drugs and banned substances such as fenfluramine in imported medicines.

This does not mean that all, or even most, Chinese medicines are unsafe. But because of the weak UK regulatory regime – and the ease of importing small quantities of medicines via postal systems or personal luggage – there is no entirely reliable way of telling which are safe, or which practitioners are properly trained. Please do not risk buying herbs or remedies from high street Chinese medicine shops and never, ever buy any sort of medicine over the internet or by mail order. Recommendations based upon personal experience can be particularly helpful. Find a registered practitioner – the Association of Traditional Chinese Medicine and Acupuncture UK (www.atcm.co.uk) is the largest regulatory body in the UK for the practice of TCM.

The MHRA publishes regular safety updates on its website, where you will also find detailed advice for patients about herbal and Chinese medicines: mhra.gov.uk.

Energy therapies

Energy therapies are based on the idea that each one of us has special energy that moves within our body or around it and that manipulating this energy can be beneficial. While none of these therapies are proven, patients say they help them to relax, improve energy levels and deal with stress and anxiety.

Healing or spiritual healing

Healers believe they act as a channel through which the healing energy that exists around each of us reaches the patient. It is often, although not necessarily, associated with a spiritual philosophy or religion. In the Christian tradition, it may be accompanied by prayer and what is called the *laying on of hands*. Each such session may last up to an hour.

Reflexology

In a reflexology session, which usually lasts 30–40 minutes, pressure is applied to areas on your feet, or occasionally your hands. Reflexologists believe these areas correspond to specific organs within the body and that the manipulation of the right area on the foot or hand will affect the organ it corresponds with. Reflexology may be used to relieve symptoms such as nausea, fatigue and pain and although there is no evidence that it is effective, it has been shown to help relaxation. Many people report they find it helpful in dealing with stress and anxiety.

Reiki

Reiki is a Japanese word that translates as *universal life energy*. It is believed to have originated in Tibet more than 2,500 years ago. During a Reiki session, the practitioner places his or her hands in 12 to 15 positions on or above parts of the patient's clothed body holding them in place for two to five minutes each. The hands are intended to be a conduit for *life energy*, balancing it within and around the body. A session usually lasts 30–60 minutes. Practitioners believe this will help release the body's natural healing powers. Reiki healing may also be practised from a distance.

Shiatsu

A Japanese form of massage based on the traditional Chinese belief that good health depends on the circulation of energy along meridians within the body. Practitioners use their fingers and thumbs to apply pressure to specific points along these meridians. They may also use other techniques such as stretching, joint rotations and rocking. A session usually lasts 45–60 minutes. Massage of any sort may not be advisable following surgery or during certain cancer treatments, so check with your medical team before you embark on shiatsu treatments.

Herbal medicine

Herbal medicines can be as powerful as pharmaceutical medicines. In fact, many modern medicines are based on the active components found in plants traditionally used in herbal medicine. The classic example is aspirin where the active ingredient is derived from salicylic acid, found in the bark of willow trees. It is often believed that because herbal medicines are 'natural' or 'plant-based' they must be safe. That is simply not true. Think of poisons like hemlock and deadly nightshade. So take care. If you want to try herbal medicines, go to a reputable herbalist. If herbal treatments are powerful enough to have an effect, they are also powerful enough to have side effects so you need advice from an expert practitioner. If they are not powerful and not effective then you have wasted your money. Do not take herbal medicines you have bought over the counter while you are having cancer treatment. They may be mild but there is still a possibility of interactions.

Even herbal medicines that are generally safe can interfere unpredictably with the action of your cancer drugs. They might increase or decrease their actions, affect your blood pressure or cause toxicity. A reputable herbalist will offer to contact your oncologist to discuss your treatment. Although a surprising number of conventional doctors will agree to collaborate, many oncologists ask patients to avoid any herbal medicine during treatment. If this is your experience, you can at least ask them about using ginger to relieve nausea and camomile tea to help relaxation and sleep as they may see no problem with these.

Surgery and herbal medicines

Tell your doctors about any herbal medicines you are taking if you are due to have surgery as some can interfere with blood pressure. They may also interfere with anaesthetics, anti-coagulants and other medications used before, during and after surgery. Some herbal medicines build up within the body over time, so you may be advised to give them up several weeks before your surgery. If you are considering Chinese, Ayurveda or any other ethnic herbal medicines, please read the warning on page 92.

The law and herbal medicine

An EU Directive passed in 2011 banned the sale of unlicensed herbal remedies, and herbal medicines are now only available from registered healthcare practitioners who are members of a regulated profession. In February 2011, the UK government promised to introduce a regulatory system for medical herbalists and practitioners of Traditional Chinese Medicine so that the public could access herbal medicines safely if they wished to do so. However, at the time of writing, no action has been taken and some scientists and medical organisations have lobbied the government to ban herbal medicine altogether.

For the time being, medical herbalists are being allowed to practise but it is unclear for how long. They can make up prescriptions on their own premises but are no longer allowed to purchase from so-called 'third-party suppliers', small specialist laboratories which make up herbal prescriptions to stringent safety and quality standards. Many have gone out of business as a result of the EU Directive and some herbalists have stopped practising. Herbal medicine may disappear within the next few years, or even be banned.

Herbal medicines on sale over the counter direct to the public have to be licensed either with a full product licence like any other medicine or through the Traditional Herbal Registration (THR) system. Some may have slipped through the safety net so always check the back of the package for the licence number which will begin with either PL (for 'product licence') or THR.

Under the THR scheme, manufacturers do not have to provide proof that their products work but they must ensure that they meet quality and safety standards. The products have to be described as based on 'traditional use' and intended to treat only minor conditions that are suitable for self-care. Some scientists and doctors have criticised this scheme, saying that all medicines should have to provide proof of efficacy on the basis of scientific, double-blind, randomised controlled trials. We disagree because there are other good types of evidence for a product's efficacy.[11]

For more information about herbal medicine, including TCM and Ayurveda, contact the European Herbal and Traditional Medicine Practitioners Association: www.ehpa.eu or email info@ehpa.eu; or visit the National Institute of Medical Herbalists website at nimh.org.uk.

Research into herbal medicines and cancer

There are hundreds of herbal medicines, some based on single plants (or parts of a plant) and others on combinations. A small number have been investigated for anti-cancer effects and some positive evidence has been found.

- **Artemisinin**, extracted from wormwood and best known for its anti-malarial effects has been shown to inhibit cancer proliferation, metastasis and angionesis in laboratory studies. In xenograft animal models, exposure to artemisinin substantially reduced the volume of the tumour and progression of the cancer.[12]
- **Blue-green algae** has been shown to increase the level of natural killer cells circulating in blood and thus boost immunity in studies on healthy humans. Spirulina, a commonly available type of blue-green alga, is sold in health food shops. Certain blue-green algae and Madagascan periwinkle contain chemicals that act on the sodium-ion channels found in individual cells (see page 34). However, one compound found in periwinkle is toxic and many herbalists will not use it for that reason.
- **Mistletoe** is widely used in herbal medicine. The extracts from the berries and shoots contain a range of active ingredients including lectins, viscotoxins, oligosaccharides and polysaccharides. These can help activate the body's natural killer cells and increase the activity of the immune system. In animals, mistletoe extracts, or substances like triterpene contained in mistletoe shoots, can produce potent anti-tumour effects.[13] Several clinical studies of mistletoe therapy on a range of cancers have shown that its use may help improve survival, increase the length of time before the cancer recurs, improve quality of life and enable a reduction in the dose – and side effects – of conventional treatments.[14] However, mistletoe can interfere with the action of some chemotherapy or drugs like steroids and cyclosporine which are commonly used after bone-marrow and stem-cell transplants. This herb can also increase the effects of some drugs used to treat high blood pressure. You must inform your oncologist if you intend to use mistletoe extracts during your treatment.

- **Mushrooms** have immunotherapeutic properties that can be useful against cancer. It doesn't apply to all mushrooms, but shiitake is just one variety that may help fight the development and progression of cancer. Mushrooms can be potent stimulators of natural killer cells and macrophages – white blood cells which protect the body against infections.[15] The active ingredients of the mushrooms mainly responsible for this effect are beta-glucans, proteins which are thought to bind to specific receptors on the immune cells and stimulate them. Remember, however, that several species of mushroom are poisonous or can induce psychosis, so never eat mushrooms you have picked in the wild.

Homeopathy

Although homeopathy is extremely popular, it is difficult to defend scientifically and has recently been the subject of great controversy. Currently, there are three NHS homeopathic hospitals (see box on page 101) but some leading doctors and scientists argue that it should not be provided on the NHS. In 2013, England's Chief Medical Officer described homeopathy as 'rubbish'.

How is it supposed to work?

Homeopathy is based on the idea that 'like treats like'. For example, something that irritates the bladder may be used to treat cystitis. Also certain substances taken in minuscule amounts will cure the same symptoms it would cause if taken in large amounts. Homeopathic medicines are made by repeatedly diluting and *succussing* (shaking) the original preparation in water and alcohol. Each dilution involves adding one part of the original substance to 99 parts of water. After dilution, the medicine may be added to small lactose tablets. Most homeopathic medicines are 6c or 30c potency – in other words the original substance has undergone a series of six or 30 dilutions. The higher the number of dilutions, the more potent the medicine is believed to be. This sounds like nonsense, but there are a small number of conventional drugs and some other chemicals that have a similarly paradoxical effect at low doses – but not if the final preparation does not contain a single molecule of the active substance, as is claimed for very high potency homeopathic remedies. Although remedies below 24c do contain some molecules of the original substance, those of 24c or higher are so dilute that they may have none left. Homeopaths believe that the water they have been diluted with somehow retains an 'imprint' or 'memory' of the original substance and that the succussing action is crucial to creating this. It is this theory that causes conventional scientists real concern. There is no real scientific evidence that this is possible, and there is no scientific theory to explain it.

Despite all this, some conventional doctors are trained in homeopathy and many people, including some cancer patients, say it has successfully treated symptoms such as nausea and fatigue. Breast-cancer patients suffering from menopausal symptoms like hot flushes, which can be made worse by taking the drug tamoxifen, say that homeopathy has helped relieve their symptoms. Homeopathy has also been used successfully to treat psychological symptoms such as depression and anxiety. It is safe and does not interact with conventional drugs and therapies.

The evidence

The British Homeopathic Association, which represents doctors and healthcare professionals who are also qualified in homeopathy, claims that clinical research has produced positive evidence for the effects of homeopathy over and above what could be expected from placebo. In 40 per cent of 163 published randomised control trials, there was a balance of positive evidence for homeopathy. Just over half were inconclusive and 7 per cent had a balance of negative evidence. Additionally, research on human cultured breast-cancer cells at the world-famous MD Anderson Cancer Center (USA)[16] showed that ultra-diluted doses of four homeopathic agents had biological activity, including delaying or arresting the process of cell division and triggering apoptosis – programmed cell death – in cancer cells.

However, none of these trials have produced incontrovertible evidence that homeopathy works. Homeopaths, and many other complementary practitioners, say that RCTs used to assess the efficacy of conventional medicines are not the ideal way of testing their treatments. RCTs test the same medicine on a group of patients who all have the same condition. However, in homeopathy, the medicine is tailored for each individual patient,

Homeopathy on the NHS

There are three small homeopathic NHS hospitals which all now provide a range of complementary treatments integrated with conventional care.

- The Royal London Hospital for Integrated Medicine is part of the University College Hospitals NHS Foundation Trust which only treats outpatients and accepts referrals from around the country. All its clinics are led by NHS consultants, doctors and other healthcare professionals.
- The Bristol Homeopathic Hospital is part of the University Hospitals Bristol NHS Trust and provides a Complementary Cancer Care service, again led by NHS consultants. Patients are normally seen within four to eight weeks of referral.
- The Glasgow Homeopathic Hospital is a purpose-built and award-winning 15-bed hospital incorporating a therapy garden. It is part of NHS Greater Glasgow and Clyde.

If you want more information about homeopathy or would like to find a qualified practitioner, visit the British Homeopathic Association's website (www.britishhomeopathic.org).

taking into account the patient's lifestyle, emotional condition, diet, personality and medical history as well as their medical condition. The final prescription is likely to be a complex blend of several remedies and differs from patient to patient even though they may, in the eyes of conventional medicine, have the same condition. It is this personalised approach that appeals to many people. They are treated holistically rather than as just bodies where something broken has to be fixed.

The bottom line is that although homeopathy is difficult to defend on a purely scientific basis, some doctors and many patients believe that it can be helpful and provide effective symptom relief without being unduly dangerous when used alone. It is not known whether homeopathy could interfere with conventional medication.

Mind-body therapies

Mind-body therapies are based on the belief that what goes on in the mind affects the body. This belief is backed up by brain-scanning studies that have shown how different emotional states directly affect the brain, triggering a cascade of chemical changes that can, in turn, influence organs and tissues throughout the body.[17] Historically, this field has suffered from poorly designed research, but more recent well-designed studies provide convincing evidence of the benefits of mind-body techniques in supporting cancer treatment. An increasing number of patients have been using these techniques to help manage the emotional stress associated with cancer. They may have other benefits as well – reduced pain, anxiety, insomnia, anticipatory and treatment-related nauseas, hot flushes, and improved mood. Importantly, the research shows that the positive effects of mind-body treatments are not psychological or some kind of placebo.

Mind-body therapies are available in many cancer centres – often almost regarded as part of the conventional healthcare package – helping patients to reduce their anxiety, sleep better and ease pain or other side effects. They must be practised regularly to get results.

Creative therapies

Art, music and writing therapies are used to help people express themselves and communicate their feelings. They are approved for use within the NHS, but provision is thin in some areas. Arts therapists – who work with the visual arts, music and drama – are registered healthcare professionals whose status is equivalent to dietitians, speech and language therapists and similar professions allied to medicine. Some are also qualified psychotherapists.

Hypnotherapy

During hypnosis, the therapist leads you into a deeply relaxed trance state. You remain aware of your surroundings at all times but the predominant feeling is one of comfortable relaxation. It is believed that in this state your unconscious mind is open to suggestions from the therapist that enable you to make beneficial life changes. Hypnosis cannot make anyone do anything they do not want to do and you cannot be hypnotised against your will. Hypnosis has been shown to help in controlling pain, reducing nausea and improving well-being. One recent study in the USA found that women given hypnotherapy before surgery for breast cancer experienced less pain, nausea and anxiety.[18] Another found that hot flushes were reduced and less severe in women who had hypnosis following surgery.[19] A large review found evidence that children undergoing cancer treatment experienced less pain and distress if treated with hypnotherapy.[20]

Hynotherapy is generally safe and does not interact with conventional treatments. However, people with some mental health conditions should not use it because it could make them worse and anyone with epilepsy should check with their doctor. Take care when choosing your therapist as there is no legal training requirement or single professional body. Most doctors, clinical psychologists and other healthcare professionals who practise it are members of the **British Society of Clinical Hypnosis** (www.bsch.org.uk).

Meditation

Meditation is an important part of Eastern religions as well as some Christian traditions but you do not have to be religious to meditate. Although it can take time to learn and experience its benefits, studies have shown that it can reduce blood pressure, boost the immune system, reduce stress and control symptoms such as pain and sickness. A recent study which used Magnetic Resonance Imaging (MRI) showed that meditators had significantly higher thresholds for pain[21] which was related to changes in the regions of brain concerned with pain signalling, implying that long-term meditation practice led to structural changes in the brain.[22] As well as group classes and one-to-one teachers, there are many books and CDs to help you learn how to meditate.

Mindfulness is a form of meditation that originated in Buddhist practice which involves becoming aware of and focusing on the present moment. Like meditation, mindfulness practice has been shown to lower pain sensitivity.[23]

A recent development is Mindfulness Based Stress Reduction (MBSR) which is now being used to treat a range of clinical conditions, including stress and anxiety in cancer patients. It usually involves an eight-week course where you are taught techniques to enable you to become aware of and focus on the present moment. It may include a sitting meditation, focusing on breathing and consciously experiencing the sensations in your own body – even your thoughts – then moving on to mindful movement and walking mindfulness. Ask your medical team if it is provided by your local hospital or available privately, although this can be expensive, costing up to £300–£400 for an eight-week course. Other courses based at Sangha centres cost much less. You can find details of these centres on the internet.

Relaxation techniques

Relaxation is a benefit of many complementary therapies, but you may also be given the opportunity to learn simple relaxation techniques without undertaking a more complex therapy such as meditation. Breathing exercises and other gentle techniques can help relieve tension and stress. Books and CDs are widely available, as well as group classes.

Visualisation

Along with relaxation, this is one of the most popular therapies among cancer patients. You will be asked to adopt a comfortable position and relax as much as possible. The therapist then guides you through imagining a peaceful scene such as lying on a beach or in a flower-filled meadow where you feel healthy and strong. You use all your senses – sight, touch, smell, hearing and even taste. The idea behind it is that you can use your imagination to help produce physical change, for instance to improve your sleep or deal with symptoms and side effects. It is possible to learn visualisation alone from books or CDs, but to start with you are likely to find guided visualisation more helpful.

A number of studies suggest it can be effective, although the results are not conclusive. For instance, recent US research involving women having radiotherapy for breast cancer found that those who practised guided visualisation had lower blood pressure, pulse and breathing rates than those who did not.[24] They also had a slightly higher skin temperature, showing they were more relaxed.[25]

Psychological and talking therapies

Being told that you have cancer is life changing and can have a massive psychological effect. Just coping with the symptoms and treatment takes its toll. It is hardly surprising that anxiety and depression are common, and that many people begin to question their basic assumptions and beliefs. Psychological and talking therapies can provide much-needed support at this time.

Cognitive Behaviour Therapy

Cognitive behaviour therapy (CBT) is a talking therapy that aims to help you manage problems by looking at the way you think and behave. It is widely used and generally regarded as effective. You may be offered one-to-one sessions with a CBT-trained therapist or clinical psychologist. Alternatively, some centres offer weekly group sessions.

CBT has been studied as a treatment for insomnia and pain in patients with a range of cancers and was found to be more effective than standard treatments, usually sleeping pills or other medication.[26] The patients who took part in the study also reported less tiredness, anxiety and depression than those who did not receive CBT.

Counselling

People with cancer can feel as though their emotions are in complete turmoil. It can be difficult to talk to family and friends when you feel bewildered and often frightened as well. A trained counsellor can help you make sense of your reactions and emotions, and help you find a way of coping with them. Counselling may be available through your NHS cancer centre or via your GP practice. **Macmillan Cancer Support** (www.macmillan.org.uk) can also give details of counsellors in your local area.

Group therapy

Many people find sharing their experience with other cancer patients in a group situation both helpful and supportive. The sessions are led by a trained therapist who guides the discussion. Studies show that group therapy can improve well-being and quality of life. There is even some preliminary research that suggests it can delay the development of secondary cancers and extend life. Your care team will be able to tell you about group therapy opportunities in your area.

You can get details of counsellors and psychotherapists in your area from the British Association for Counselling and

Psychotherapy (www.bacp.co.uk). Maggie's Centres across the UK provide support for anyone affected by cancer. Among other services they offer two six-week programmes: *Living with Cancer* (for those with a diagnosis); *Caring for Someone with Cancer* (for partners and other relatives). You can find out more about **Maggie's Centres** and their services at www.maggiescentres.org

Touch and massage therapies

The idea that touch can be healing is truly ancient and massage is possibly the oldest therapy known to man. Research has confirmed that touch therapies can help with psychological symptoms associated with cancer and also with some physical problems.

Aromatherapy

Aromatherapy involves the use of *essential oils* – natural oils extracted from plants that are thought to have specific healing properties. These are diluted in a neutral carrier such as almond oil and generally massaged into the body. Alternatively, a few drops can be placed in your bath or used in diffusers. Different oils are said to have different effects. For instance, lavender is known for its relaxing effect whereas rosemary is believed to be invigorating. Studies into the effectiveness of specific oils have been inconclusive, but patients report an improvement in their well-being, mood and stress levels.

As well as whole-body treatments, many people find neck and shoulder or hand massage with aromatherapy oils pleasant and relaxing. These can be given without the need to take your clothes off. Aromatherapy may be provided free of charge in NHS hospitals and many nurses and midwives have learnt the technique. If you are thinking about having aromatherapy treatment privately, always make sure your therapist is properly trained and has experience dealing with cancer patients. Your cancer nurse may be able to advise you about local practitioners. Alternatively check the register maintained by the **Complementary and Natural Healthcare Council** (www.cnhc.org.uk).

Massage

Massage has been shown to relax the mind, help with sleeping, relieve tension and stress, and improve the circulation of blood and lymph. There are many different types of massage therapy, some gentle and others more vigorous and perhaps uncomfortable. People with cancer are advised to choose the more gentle types and to make sure their therapist is properly trained and experienced in treating cancer patients. It is important not to apply deep pressure to areas of the body that are near the cancer or being treated with radiotherapy, around catheters or any area that has been affected by blood clots. If cancer has spread to the bones it is particularly important to be gentle. Some people worry that massage might encourage cancer to spread but there is no evidence of this happening. People who bruise or bleed easily should check with their doctor before having massage.

Vitamin C injection

The idea of using antioxidants as complementary therapy for cancer has been under discussion for many years. On the one hand, antioxidants can protect against the potentially damaging effects of free radicals. However, this is also precisely how some treatments, like chemotherapy and radiotherapy, are meant to kill cancer cells. Not surprisingly, therefore, both beneficial and harmful effects of antioxidant use in cancer have been reported. Remember that diet is very important (Step 5) so a lot can be done to improve your body's chemistry through your eating habits. Nevertheless, there is one antioxidant supplement worthy of consideration – vitamin C!

The idea of using vitamin C (ascorbic acid) against cancer came from the eminent chemist and double Nobel Prize winner, Linus Pauling, in the 1970s. Its potential success is based upon two characteristics of vitamin C. First, it is a potent antioxidant. Second, it is soluble in water and not in fat so it cannot accumulate in the body and any excess will be extruded in urine. Studies have shown that, to be effective, vitamin C should be injected intravenously rather than taken orally. Vitamin C is safe even at high concentrations (up to 10,000 mg daily). A study on mice with a type of tumour called a sarcoma showed that those who received a high dose of vitamin C, injected into their body cavity, survived about 20 per cent longer than untreated animals; the increased survival was through inhibition of angiogenesis (the development of blood vessels, which feed the tumour).[27] The effects of vitamin C injections combined with chemotherapy were also tested on humans. One study on breast-cancer patients showed that intravenous vitamin C administration resulted in a significant reduction in quality-of-life-related side effects resulting from the cancer, chemotherapy and radiotherapy.[28] Also, another, small-scale (phase I) study on stage IV pancreatic-cancer patients showed (a) that adding vitamin C to the chemotherapy drugs gemcitabine and erlotinib did not result in increased toxicity and (b) seven of the nine subjects who completed the treatment regimen had stable disease; this justified longer-term (phase II) trials.[29] Another study on ovarian-cancer patients where intravenous vitamin C was used in combination with chemotherapy found that it significantly reduced the adverse side effects from the drug regime.[30] Several other clinical trials are ongoing and will show if vitamin C injections can directly shrink tumours.

Returning to the issue of antioxidants in general, the balance of advantage-disadvantage may vary from antioxidant to antioxidant, the type of cancer and its ongoing treatment. The bottom line is that the kind of natural diet that we have recommended in Step 5 is best to follow and will ensure that 'antioxidants' are consumed in healthy balance.

Therapies to avoid

The treatments below are often advertised on websites targeted at cancer patients. They do not work, will not help you recover from cancer and will probably cost you a great deal of money.

Some should carry a safety warning as they may be harmful. We have listed several of these therapies below but want to emphasise that this list is not exhaustive and new 'therapies to avoid' will continue to appear. So, we advise extreme caution.

Essiac tea

This tea is a mixture of herbs – originally, burdock root, slippery elm inner bark, sheep sorrel and Indian rhubarb, with watercress, blessed thistle, red clover and kelp added later. It was invented by a Canadian nurse, René Caisse ('Essiac' is 'Caisse' spelt backwards) who thought that it would reduce tumour growth by cleaning the blood, disposing of tissue by-products and enhancing the body's innate defence mechanisms.

Research into the supposed anti-cancer effects of Essiac was carried out in 1959 and again in the 1970s. The renowned Memorial Sloan-Kettering Cancer Centre conducted some initial animal tests but found no anti-cancer effect. Further studies reached the same conclusion. No major medical or scientific organisation that we are aware of (including the FDA, the NCI and the American Cancer Society) support the anti-cancer claims made by the Essiac promoters. Apart from a possible placebo effect, it seems that Essiac tea is unlikely to help.[31] Some non-serious side effects have been reported such as increased bowel movements, frequent urination, swollen glands, skin blemishes, flu-like symptoms and slight headaches. It is not clear if Essiac might interact with other drugs.

Germanium (and Germanium 132)

Germanium is a potentially harmful treatment, widely available over the internet, which – at first glance – seems to have some theoretical evidence to support it. Germanium is a type of chemical element called a 'metalloid' used commonly as a semi-conductor in electronic components. It is toxic and not suitable for human or animal consumption. However, it also exists in a non-toxic organic form in very small amounts in some plant-based foods – much like iron or calcium which occur naturally in foods like ginseng, garlic, shiitake mushrooms and rhubarb.

Germanium 132 (Ge 132; bis-carboxyethyl germanium sesquioxide) is a synthetic substance that is similar to natural, organic germanium. It is a powerful antioxidant and theoretically might be able to boost the body's immune system by encouraging the creation of white blood cells. However, germanium products – sold as medicines or health foods – may contain toxic inorganic germanium. Lack of regulation means that it is not possible to know what you are buying and germanium 'medicines' which contain inorganic germanium have been reported to cause kidney damage, sleep disruption or mental disturbance. A number of deaths have also been reported.[32]

Gerson therapy

Gerson practitioners believe that fertilisers, pesticides and other chemicals contaminate food and change the metabolism of our cells, eventually causing cancer.[33] The therapy requires patients to follow a strict low-salt, low-fat, vegetarian diet, drinking the juice of about 20 pounds (9 kilograms) of fresh fruits and vegetables a day. They are given frequent coffee enemas, and supplements, such as potassium, vitamin B12, pancreatic enzymes, thyroid hormone, and liver extracts, to stimulate organ function. Other supplements such as laetrile (apricot kernels) may be recommended. Critics, including the American Cancer Society,[34] point out that not only are there no studies showing that the Gerson therapy is effective, but also that the regime can lead to serious illness. For example, coffee enemas could lead to electrolyte imbalances and may over time cause the colon's normal function to weaken, worsening constipation and colitis. They add that infections may result from poorly administered liver extracts, and thyroid supplements may cause severe bleeding in patients whose cancer has spread to the liver. The most serious criticism, however, is that practitioners can advise patients to rely on the Gerson therapy alone and avoid conventional medical treatment. Undoubtedly that advice is of serious concern. We believe it is frankly dangerous.

Gonzalez regimen

This is a complex treatment plan that is supposed to fight cancer by helping the body eliminate toxins (from the environment and processed foods). The aim is to keep the immune system healthy and balance the part of the nervous system that controls automatic body functions such as heartbeat, blood pressure, digestion and breathing. Its developer, Dr Nicholas Gonzalez, promotes it as a treatment for advanced pancreatic cancer. The treatment involves taking a freeze-dried pancreatic enzyme obtained from pigs, said to be the main cancer-fighter in the regime. Patients also take a large number of nutritional supplements, including magnesium citrate, papaya, vitamins and other minerals; eat a special diet of mainly organic foods; and take coffee enemas.

There is no evidence that this treatment is effective against cancer and it is not approved by any major medical or scientific organisation. An extensive clinical study on pancreatic cancer patients, reported in the peer-reviewed *Journal of Clinical Oncology* in 2010, concluded that the Gonzalez regimen provided no relative advantage. In fact, patients treated with chemotherapy alone reported a better quality of life and survived longer.[35]

Hoxsey treatment

This therapy, developed in the first half of the 20th century, originally involved two herbal mixtures. A paste or powder containing antimony, zinc and bloodroot, arsenic, sulphur and talc, to be rubbed directly onto tumours, and a liquid tonic, containing licorice, red clover, burdock root, Stillingia root, barberry, Cascara, prickly ash bark, buckthorn bark and potassium iodide, for internal consumption. The treatment now also involves antiseptic douches and washes, laxative tablets and nutritional supplements. A mixture of procaine hydrochloride and vitamins, along with liver and cactus is also prescribed. There is no scientific basis for any of these concoctions. Food restrictions are part of the treatment as well – patients are asked to avoid consumption of tomatoes, vinegar, pork, alcohol, salt, sugar, and white-flour products. Reviews by major medical bodies, including the FDA, the National Cancer Institute, the American Cancer Society, MD Anderson Cancer Center and Memorial Sloan-Kettering Cancer Center found no evidence that Hoxsey treatment has any effect against cancer. The paste or powder can severely burn, scar and disfigure the skin and although it is not clear whether the liquid tonic is dangerous, some of the individual ingredients can have side effects including nausea, diarrhoea and vomiting and may interact with other drugs. The sale or marketing of the Hoxsey method in the USA was banned by the FDA in 1960. Again in 2008, the FDA emphasised the complete lack of evidence and credibility for the Hoxsey method.[36] Nevertheless, it is still marketed over the internet and at the time of writing was practised by the Bio-Medical Center in Tijuana, Mexico.

Hyperbaric oxygen therapy

Although hyperbaric oxygen (HBO) therapy is used in conventional cancer care to treat severe side effects, particularly those from radiation therapy, it does not destroy cancer cells and is not a cancer treatment in its own right – yet that is how some private clinics promote it. Their argument is that because cancer thrives in a low-oxygen environment, immersing the cancer in oxygen can kill it. This misunderstands the nature of how cancer cells metabolise. As we saw in Step 1, cancer cells generate their energy from a natural chemical called glycogen rather than using oxygen as normal cells do. Importantly, it does not matter how much oxygen is available, the cancer will always use glycogen instead of oxygen. Furthermore, scientific evidence shows that oxygen dissolved in blood cannot enter cancers so effectively because of their disorderly and poorly developed blood vessels.[37]

This treatment is both time consuming and expensive. If you are offered HBO therapy as part of your conventional NHS treatment, you might wish to accept as it may not harm. But do not waste money or time on it as 'alternative' treatment at private clinics: your valuable time would be better spent in getting effective treatment from a good oncologist and medical team.

Misuse of PDT

Photodynamic therapy (PDT) is a relatively new, still-developing treatment that is licensed for the treatment of some cancers, as we described in Step 3. The patient is given photosensitive chemicals, which are taken up by cancer cells, and targeted light is then used to destroy the cancer. Although it is effective in early-stage lung cancer, oesophageal cancer and Bowen's disease, PDT only has limited uses and cancer patients can be exploited by private clinics here and abroad. The main reason is that light simply will not penetrate more than 1 centimetre below the skin. In conventional treatment, as used in the NHS, an endoscope is used to access deeper tumours. Private clinics rarely do this – instead they put the patient into a tent or tank which allows the body to be bathed in (usually red) light which is likely to be useless because the light will not reach the cancer.

You might also see internet advertisements for so-called 'advanced' versions of PDT, called 'next-generation PDT' (NGPDT) from clinics based in the UK, Mexico, China and elsewhere. These are not supported by scientific evidence and have been criticised for falsely claiming that these therapies can treat late-stage cancers. Medical experts criticial of these clinics believe that the people running them are misguided at best or, at worst, downright fraudulent. The treatment usually is very expensive, and you could be putting your life at risk by having NGPDT rather than following NHS advice or treatment. Your condition may deteriorate further and you may experience unknown adverse effects from the therapy. These treatments are not even suitable as a last resort for incurable cancer as they may result in unnecessary pain,[38] see http://www.nhs.uk/Conditions/photodynamic-therapy-NGPDT-sonodynamic-therapy/Pages/Introduction.aspx.

Protocel (also called Cancell or Cantrol)
Developed in the USA in the 1950s by chemist James Sheridan, Protocel is thought to contain a cocktail of chemicals, including inositol, nitric acid, sodium sulphite, potassium hydroxide, sulphuric acid, catechol, crocinic acid and various minerals and vitamins, although the precise contents are unknown. According to the USA Food and Drug Administration, none of these have any worthwhile anti-cancer effects. The National Cancer Institute (NCI) has also dismissed it (see http://www.cancer.gov/cancertopics/pdq/cam/cancell/HealthProfessional). Since 1989 it has been illegal for the manufacturers to send Protocel across USA State lines.

Interestingly, Protocel is said to have been 'designed' to selectively target cells that generate their energy from glycogen instead of oxygen – essentially all cancer cells, as we discussed in Step 1. Protocel's main manufacturers claim that the mixture has been used by thousands of patients and that it is safe and effective in treating 50–80 per cent of cancers. However, these findings have not been published in peer-reviewed scientific journals, no clinical trials of Protocel have been reported and their only evidence is patient testimonials and anecdotal reports. In short, there is no acceptable, credible scientific basis for claims that Protocel or any of its components can target and treat cancer selectively or effectively. Nevertheless, Protocel has vast exposure on the internet and we know from personal contacts that patients are still using it as an anti-cancer agent. The treatment may cause fatigue and nausea – but more worryingly patients may be encouraged to abandon their conventional treatment in favour of a treatment that has no credible scientific evidence behind it.

Shark cartilage

Shark cartilage is sold as a dietary supplement in many health food shops and has been widely touted as an alternative treatment for cancer. Using animal parts to fight disease has always been popular in folk medicine, especially in Africa and the Far East, but without any real evidence that it works. Sharks caught the attention of the marine biologist Lawrence Barton when he noticed they never seemed to form tumours. Furthermore, the fact that cartilage does not contain blood vessels raised the possibility that it might contain some anti-angiogenic factors, and biochemical analyses suggested that this might be the case. Although some laboratory experiments showed that shark cartilage extracts had some anti-cancer effects, repeated animal tests and clinical trials on patients have failed to show that it is effective against cancer.[39]

This kind of discrepancy between positive laboratory findings and negative results from animal and human trials is not uncommon. Although the reason for such discrepancies is not always clear, what is clear is that there is currently no scientific or medical evidence that shark cartilage can fight cancer. Although side effects are rare they can include nausea, vomiting, diarrhoea, constipation, loss of appetite, fatigue, low blood pressure, dizziness and high blood calcium levels. Taking shark cartilage may also slow down the healing process for people recovering from surgery.

where do you go from here?

Clearly, 'complementary therapy' is a minefield (as well as big business), which can leave you confused and exposed! On the one hand, there are a few therapies, like acupuncture, that are proven to be effective in alleviating some of the side effects of cancer and its treatment. Then, there are those therapies for which there is neither clinical evidence nor scientific basis, like homeopathy, that patients want to use and may even derive some benefit from. In both cases there is little information about the possible consequences of combination with conventional treatment. Worst of all, there are those procedures that are useless and even dangerous and these must be avoided at all cost.

There can be no doubt that complementary therapy will continue to make an impact in the cancer field. At present, as well as for the future, we recommend caution. Remember the three questions you should ask yourself in evaluating initially any such procedure on the internet (see page 86). Remember also that cancer is best treated by multidisciplinary teams in hospital and we can hope that complementary therapists will be a part of that in the years to come. Although Western-style medical training currently does little in this area, you should still let your team know if you are intending to take any 'supplement' or undergo any complementary procedure.

step 5
eat to beat cancer

It may be a cliché that you are what you eat, but there are few areas where it rings truer than when it comes to cancer development and prevention. The links between diet and cancer were highlighted more than 30 years ago when Professors Richard Doll and Richard Peto reported that more than a third of all cancers might be attributable to dietary factors.[1] Since then it has become clear that diet plays a role in preventing as well as increasing the risk of a whole range of cancers – for example, research suggests that around 90 per cent of colorectal cancers may be preventable through changes in diet.[2] More recently, the distinguished nutritional biochemist Professor T. Colin Campbell of Cornell University has shown that the right diet prevents many common cancers, and that diet may also be the key to turning on – and turning off – existing cancers.[3]

Numerous scientific studies[4] have shown not only that the risk of developing cancer is related to your diet, but that people who eat more animal foods are more vulnerable to a range of cancers than those whose diet contains more fruit, vegetables and other plant-based foods. There is in fact a direct relationship between the incidences of many cancers and the amount of animal-based food that we eat, whereas there is no relationship with the amount of plant-based food we consume (Figure 5.1, page 133).[5]

Recent studies link a wide range of cancers, including colorectal,[6] oesophageal,[7] bladder,[8] breast, prostate,[9] gastric,[10] ovarian,[11] kidney and even pancreatic cancer,[12] to high intakes of animal foods, especially processed meat and dairy. High-fat dairy was strongly implicated in two types of oesophageal cancer.[13] Recent research found that women with the most plant-based diets were 3.5 times less likely to be diagnosed with pre-cancerous cervical lesions than women whose diets contained more meat, fat and junk food.[14] The same study also showed that a plant-based diet lowers the risk of head and neck and bladder cancer as well as pre-cancerous conditions such as colorectal adenomas.

In another study published in 2014, high levels of animal protein in the diet of middle-aged people (under 65) have also been shown to increase the risk of death from cancer or diabetes fourfold, and almost double the risk of dying generally. The overall harmful effects were almost eliminated when the protein came from plant sources, although cancer risk remained higher in middle-aged people who ate a high-protein diet.

Professor Longo, director of the Longevity Institute at the University of Southern California who led the research suggests that people should consume no more than 0.8g of protein per kilogram of body weight (about 48g for a 60kg person).

Most people in Britain eat more protein than they need. The British Dietetic Association recommends a daily intake of 55g and 45g of protein for the average man and woman respectively; however, according to the British Nutrition Foundation, the average daily protein intake is 88g and 64g for men and women.

Longo's team carried out blood tests on the people in the study. These showed that levels of IGF-1 (see page 138) tracked their protein intake. For those on a high-protein diet, rises in IGF-1 steadily increased their cancer risk. Tests on mice showed that a high-protein diet led to more and larger tumours than a low-protein diet.[15]

The food revolution

Today's Western diet is so different from the one we evolved to eat that our ancestors would hardly recognise it. For tens of millions of years our ancestors lived in small groups foraging for edible tubers, leafy plants, nuts, seeds, fruit and berries as well as hunting – and occasionally catching – animals to eat. Our closest living relatives, the chimpanzees, with which we share 99 per cent of our DNA, are predominantly herbivorous. Human beings living at low latitudes have eaten predominantly plant-based diets since prehistoric times. It was mainly as early humans migrated north that the amount of animal protein in the diet increased, a pattern that remains to this day.[16]

The latest UK national diet and nutrition survey shows that our diet is now dominated by refined cereals, (industrialised) meat, dairy and other animal products, with far less fruit and vegetables than our bodies were designed for.[17] Most dramatic of all has been the increase in fast and convenience foods and the use of additives. An estimated 3,800 chemicals – or more – are now used as additives to flavour, colour or preserve such foods and the average person in the West now eats more than 4 kg of food additives a year.[18] The book *Fast Food Nation* listed more than 50 synthetic chemicals used to make the artificial strawberry flavour in milk shakes.[19] On top of that, many chemical pesticides, introduced since the Second World War, have been found to be carcinogenic. We consider pesticides and other environmental carcinogens in more detail on pages 177–192 in Step 7.

The bottom line is that we are eating an unnatural diet, and it is not surprising that there is a price to pay. It is against this beleaguered nutritional background that many common cancers flourish.

how diet affects your cancer risk

It is becoming increasingly apparent that what we eat can directly, or indirectly, create conditions in which cancer can flourish, or alternatively provide protection so that cancer does not take hold.

At the most basic level what we eat provides us with the energy and vital nutrients that our bodies need to function. A diet that is rich in fruit and vegetables, for example, contains vitamins and plant chemicals that will help maintain a healthy immune system and may also help protect against the DNA damage that we know can happen as a result of normal metabolism.

But the role of diet is even more complex and far-reaching. Take salt, for example. In Step 1 we outlined the role of the sodium channel in cancer cells in increasing their 'excitability' and enabling them to invade other tissues – so it follows that a high-salt (sodium) diet may be significant when it comes to cancer risk.

There is also increasing evidence that diet affects the microbe population living in our intestine, known as our gut biota. Recent research on the gut microbiome (the trillions of microbes lining your small intestine, along with their interacting genes) has shown that it has many important biochemical functions in the body – and when things go wrong it can lead to disease.[20] The development of colon cancer, for example, is linked closely with a high intake of red and processed meat. New advances in sequencing technologies have given us the opportunity to study the characteristics of the human gut microbiome and the effects of what we eat – and the findings are striking. A change in diet from a low-fat, plant-based diet to a high-fat, high-sugar diet, for example, has been shown to shift the structure of our gut microbiota in a *single* day. There is much more work to be done but understanding microbiome activity is now seen as essential to the development of future personalised healthcare.

We know that cancer development also depends on the interaction between our genes and lifestyle factors, including diet

– so what you eat can actually have an impact at a genetic level. While the genes we are born with are there for life, 'bad' genes such as cancer genes do not cause problems if they are not turned on or 'expressed'. There is increasing evidence that diet is important in determining whether cancer genes are expressed or not.[21]

The power of what we do, or do not, put into our mouths was illustrated by Dean Ornish MD, Clinical Professor of Medicine at the University of California, when he showed that early-stage prostate cancer could be reversed by diet and lifestyle changes. The randomised, controlled clinical trial, conducted in collaboration with world-leading microbiologist Craig T. Venter, found that after only three months on a plant-based diet, over 450 cancer genes had been down-regulated and 48 protective genes had been up-regulated. In other words genes linked to prostate (and breast) cancer had been turned off and protective genes turned on. Patients with otherwise untreated early prostate cancer were put into remission. The diet Professor Ornish used was a vegan diet, similar to the one we have outlined in this chapter for those with active cancer (see page 125).[22]

Another recent intervention study showed that eating more fruit, vegetables and fibre and less saturated fat could help maintain lower levels of PSA (the protein which is an indicator of prostate cancer) in men who had had recurrent prostate cancer.[23] Intervention studies using diet to treat other cancers are now underway.

So cutting out the wrong foods and eating the right ones could have the potential to help stop cancer in its tracks by depriving the early-stage cancer cells – the initiated cells that we learned about in Step 1 – of the conditions they need to grow. As we learnt in Step 1, cancer cells are our own cells that have sustained damage to their DNA, particularly the 'cell cycle genes' which control cell reproduction. This damage makes them hypersensitive to tiny chemical messenger proteins called 'growth factors' that circulate in our blood. Whereas normal cells are unaffected, as another set of proteins tells them to stop, this doesn't work for cancer cells.

They 'think' they have been told to go into their reproductive cycle and hence can grow out of control.

Many scientists now believe that initiated cells are formed throughout our lives but most do not develop into active cancers. It can help to think of them as seeds that can develop into cancer only if they are given water and fertiliser.[24] The fertiliser all cancer cells need are growth-factor proteins and, in the case of hormone-dependent cancers such as breast or prostate cancer, animal hormones such as oestrogen or testosterone. This is particularly true of cancers of affluence (the division of cancers into those of affluence and those of poverty is discussed more fully in Step 1), in which the modern Western diet appears to be an important factor, but also to cancers of poverty, which include virus-induced cancers such as those caused by hepatitis.

Conventional medicine attacks and kills cancer cells, although some that are resistant to treatment can survive. But what if, as well as attacking the cancer cells directly, you can also change the environment within the body, by depriving it of the 'fertiliser' cancer cells need and by making it more hostile to cancer? It is rather like having a persistent weed in your garden. Although you attack it by digging it up, burning it and applying pesticides, it keeps coming back. But if the weed needs acid conditions and certain chemicals to grow and spread – by making the soil alkaline and cutting off the supply of chemicals the weed can no longer flourish and will die.

That is precisely what our nutritional programme, based on 10 food factors, aims to do to cancer cells. The programme we have outlined below is predominantly vegan. We recognise that the idea of switching to a fully vegan diet may feel daunting for some people – if you don't want to become fully vegan keep meat, fish and, especially, dairy foods to a minimum. Professor Dean Ornish suggests that if you are currently healthy but want to follow a diet that protects against cancer you should increase the amount of vegetables and fruit you eat, making sure you include plenty of beans, soya and other sources of plant protein. Harvard University is now recommending a similar diet. Try it. You might be surprised at how well and how full of energy you will feel – and how enjoyable this sort of diet can be.

We suggest that anyone with active cancer or at high risk of the disease follows the eating plan we have outlined below. It is the diet that Jane used to put her cancer into remission for a sixth time after it was re-diagnosed after almost 20 years in December 2011. Other people may wish to follow the main principles, but with a slightly less strict regime.

Your at-a-glance beat-cancer diet

Cut out	Replace it with
All dairy, whether from cows, sheep, goats or any other animal – and even if it is described as organic; if you have active cancer there are no half measures here	
Milk, including skimmed and semi-skimmed	Veggie milks such as almond, coconut, oat, rice or soya milk
Hard cheese	Tofu or bean curd (marinate for at least 2 hours in a sauce made from low-sodium soy sauce, ginger and chopped spring onions)
Soft or cottage cheese	Hummus
Yoghurt	Soya or coconut yoghurt. If you think you need the acidophilus bacteria buy capsules and empty their contents into warm water. Alternatively have low-sodium miso which also contains good bugs
Crème fraîche, fromage frais, cream	Coconut or soya cream
Butter and veggie margarines containing dairy	Soya spread, hummus or peanut or other nut butter or seed butter

Cut out	Replace it with
Diary ice cream	Soya or coconut ice cream (always check ingredients list for hidden dairy, such as milk or whey powder, lactose, milk solids/fats or casein
Milk chocolate	Dark chocolate
Refined and processed oils prepared using high temperature and/or pressure	Extra virgin olive oil or coconut oil for cooking; sunflower or sesame oil for salad dressings
Refined (especially white) sugar, honey and manmade sugars such as aspartame, often used in diet drinks and other products	Raw cane sugar (molasses), stevia or unrefined maple or rice syrup
Refined (especially white) bread, flour, pasta and rice	Unrefined wholegrain products
Any foods containing preservatives, colourings and artificial flavourings (often found in processed food, fizzy and fruit drinks and confectionery). Check ingredients lists and E numbers on the internet	Make your own fresh food and juices
Processed meat such as pâté or sausage	

Limit your consumption (eat organic product wherever possible)	Eat lots of (organic wherever possible)
Fresh meat	Unrefined carbs such as noodles, pasta, rice, bread or dairy-free cakes
Fish or shellfish	Beans such as broad beans, cannellini beans and butter beans, plus sprouting seeds and beans
Eggs	Nuts such as cashew, pistachio and walnuts or bottled water chestnuts, but avoid salted nuts or those roasted in monosodium glutamate

Vegan red wine, cloudy cider, diluted gin, malt whisky or vodka	Vegetables including sea vegetables such as seaweed (best bought from an Asian shop or supermarket). Choose fresh, frozen or bottled rather than tinned whenever possible
Salt (use sea salt) monosodium glutamate, sodium sulphite, baking soda	Herbs such as basil and parsley (fresh or dried) and spices such as cinnamon and turmeric
	Balsamic, cider, or white or red wine vinegar
	Fruit – choose fresh, frozen or bottled rather than tinned whenever possible
	Homemade juices – blend fruit and vegetables
Coffee	Tap water and herb teas

ten essential food factors

Food Factor 1: Eat real food

Cooking and sharing meals is an essential part of human behaviour and history. The starting point for any eating plan is to make selecting, preparing and cooking good food central to your way of life, rather than relying on pre-prepared microwaveable meals, as so many people now do. We believe this really is living dangerously; the recent scandal, where cheap horsemeat was being sold as beef, has underlined this message.

Cooking is intrinsic to being human. In fact the latest archaeological evidence suggests that cooking goes back a million years – even early man cooked his food.[25] Without cooking we would, like many animals, spend so much time eating and digesting food that there would be little time to do anything else. And although it can be helpful to eat some food raw, cooking can help make food more nutritious – some cancer protective plant chemicals, such as lycopene, are more bio-available in cooked food. Other foods that contain toxins when raw are safe when cooked, for example vegetables such as broccoli contain substances called goitrogens, which can affect the thyroid if eaten uncooked.[26] We suggest that vegetables like broccoli and cabbage should best be lightly steamed.

Pay attention to your cooking methods as well. Cooking starchy foods like potatoes at very high temperatures by frying or baking them can generate a carcinogenic chemical called acrylamide, while frying or barbecuing can generate other carcinogenic chemicals called heterocyclic amines (HCAs), especially in red meat. A high intake of red meat and HCAs has been linked to bladder-cancer risk in people genetically predisposed to this disease[27] as well as kidney cancer.[28] Also, avoiding high-temperature cooking of fish has been shown to lower prostate-cancer risk. In general, steaming, boiling or slow, low-temperature cooking are safer for all food types.

Take time to eat

If you used to do this	Now do this
Skip breakfast and grab a coffee at the station	Soak one cup of organic porridge oats in filtered water overnight, bring to the boil for two minutes, add raw molasses and a pinch of cinnamon, plus vegetable milk such as oat or soya milk. Have a glass of fresh orange juice and green tea.
For your elevenses, have a latte and keep working	Substitute juice or herbal tea with some nuts and dried fruit to nibble on. If possible, take a break of at least 20 minutes. Spend time talking to colleagues and just see how your working relationships improve.
Eat sandwiches for lunch so you can keep working	Take a lunch break of at least an hour and spend the time eating freshly made food with colleagues. Eat fresh fruit for dessert and wash down with fruit juice, or herbal tea or green tea.

In the afternoon break have a quick cuppa at your desk and keep staring at your computer screen	Take at least 20 minutes' break if your job allows you to do that – and if not, try persuading your employer that productivity would increase and absenteeism decrease by allowing regular breaks. Join colleagues over freshly brewed green tea.
Grab a prepared meal from your local supermarket on the way home and microwave it	Ensure that you have home-cooked food. If you are busy in the week, make all the meals for the week at the weekend and freeze them.
On Friday evening retire to the nearest pub with your workmates and try to get high on wine. Eat the odd salty crisp or nut	Everyone take it in turn to organise a meal at a good restaurant and have wine with your food. Good restaurants for plant-based food include Middle Eastern, Japanese, Chinese and Thai eateries.
At weekends eat out at burger or chicken bars with the kids. Eat cheese burgers or nuggets made from reconstituted chicken with fries	Train your children to eat good food and if you eat out try baked potatoes with baked beans, pizza with lots of veggies (but no cheese or chips) and peas with a small fishcake. Many Asian restaurants do takeaways but watch out for hidden dairy and fats.
Cook meat and two-vegetable meals for Sunday lunch	Make a delicious vegetable curry accompanied by organic brown rice or whole-grain rice and lots of side dishes such as chutneys and dried coconut. Involve the kids and partners in chopping vegetables and cooking.

Simple and easy changes like this will do more than improve your health. Before long, your stress levels will go down and your productivity will go up.

Food Factor 2: Eat organic

Despite thousands of column inches and numerous books devoted to 'detoxing', only a tiny minority mention the importance of eating organically. It is also surprising how few books recommending anti-cancer diets talk about organic food. We believe that, as someone whose life is affected by cancer, you should make it a priority that as much of your food as possible is organically produced.

Why eat organic?

We know that eating food contaminated by agricultural pesticides can expose our bodies to chemicals known to cause cancer and other damage and that people whose diet contains a high proportion of organic food have less pesticide exposure than those who do not.[29] You will find more detail about this in the box below.

There is evidence that pesticide residues are present in many conventionally produced foods including fruit and vegetables,[30] processed baby foods[31] and meat, eggs and milk products.[32] Although such substances may be present in only very tiny amounts, over time they may accumulate in human tissues to levels comparable to those shown to cause abnormalities in humans and

The dangers of pesticides

There is growing concern about the potential impact of persistent low levels of pesticides in food, water and the environment around us. There is mounting evidence of potential damage to humans and animals from long-term exposure, especially during foetal development, because some pesticides act as endocrine-disrupting chemicals which may interfere with the body's hormone activity.[35] Over a long period of time this could lead to reproductive malformations, increase the risk of certain hormone-related cancers,[36] neurodevelopmental defects and an increased risk of diabetes and obesity.[37] We also know that certain pesticides are able to generate a whole series of processes in the body which are identical to those involved in the development and spread of cancer.

wildlife.[33] People who consume meat, dairy products and oily fish from polluted sources are likely to be exposed to higher doses of substances like organochlorines and methyl-mercury (which build up through the food chain because they are fat soluble), than people whose diets are vegetable based.[34]

What about the cost?

Organically produced food is more expensive than non-organic food but if you follow this eating programme you will find that the extra cost will be offset by the other savings you make, for example, by cutting down or cutting out animal protein. Many people now grow their own vegetables in their garden or allotment and even if you have only a balcony you can grow veggies in bags and pots there.

If you cannot afford to switch to a totally organic diet, choose carefully. Prioritise buying organic fruit and potatoes that tend to need frequent pesticide treatments, whereas some field[38] and root vegetables[39] require less. The Pesticide Action Network say that the 10 plant foods with the heaviest pesticide residues are flour, potatoes, bread, apples, pears, grapes, strawberries, green beans, tomatoes and cucumber.[40] They recommend buying the organic equivalent of these items and eating more of the vegetables and fruits not on this list. Organic food must be produced to the UK Soil Association standard and carry its logo (see below). Remember that organic food may have been grown in animal waste, so it is vital to wash it thoroughly or blanch it quickly in boiling water like the Chinese do.

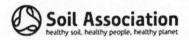

If you would like to read more about pesticides, read the chapter by McKinlay and others in the book *Pollutants, Human Health and the Environment*.[41]

Food Factor 3: Balance your diet

How often have you seen or heard the advice to eat a balanced diet? But how many people actually know what this means. We are going to show you how to balance the protein, fats and carbohydrates in your diet in a way that will really cut your cancer risk.

One of the biggest problems with the Western diet is that it contains far too much protein – especially animal protein which has been definitively linked in experimental animal studies and in epidemiological and migrant studies[42] to an increased risk of cancers such as bowel, prostate and colorectal cancers. The average adult needs only about 45–60 grams of protein a day. Many people eating a typical Western diet consume up to 16 per cent of their calories as protein – often animal protein. If they follow the recent fad for high-protein/low-carbohydrate diets, they can eat a very dangerous 20 per cent or more as protein.[43] It's not surprising that these diets have been condemned in the strongest possible terms by distinguished scientists and doctors.[44]

It is worth remembering that the primary function of protein in the body is the repair of worn-out tissues and cells. Popular high-protein/low-carb diets which rely on your body using protein rather than carbohydrate for energy[45] effectively attack the fabric of your body as it tries to create energy from the wrong fuel. This acidifies the body and can create toxic chemicals. It is like burning your furniture to warm your house instead of switching on the central-heating boiler.

By contrast in China, where until recently many types of cancer (including breast, prostate, ovary, colon and pancreatic cancer) were rare, the traditional rural diet contains only 10–11 of its calories as protein, only 1 per cent of which is animal protein. This is the ideal proportion. Exceed this and the risk of cancer goes up in a dose-dependent manner, especially if that protein is animal protein.[46] See Fig 5.1, opposite, for a comparison of the typical Chinese and Western diets.

A balanced diet looks far more like a traditional Chinese diet. Most of our daily food intake – about 70–75 per cent – should be complex, unrefined carbohydrates. These are the real fuel foods that supply energy for the brain and muscles. We also need some fats – about 15 per cent of our calories – to maintain the optimum structure and function of our brain, nerves, cell walls and some messenger molecules. Fats can also be used to generate energy. The right fats provide our bodies with effective electrical and thermal insulators but the wrong ones clog up our arteries and cause our nervous system to malfunction.

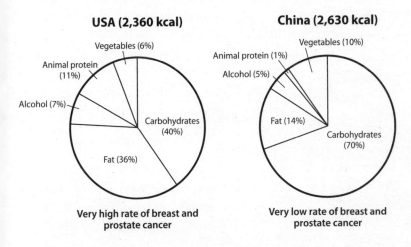

Figure 5.1. *Comparison of US and Chinese diets.*[47]

Food Factor 4: Reduce your intake of acid generating foods

The stomach is the only organ in the human body that is meant to contain acid and our bodies are naturally slightly alkaline (see page 135 for detailed information on the pH scale). However, what we eat can change this. If we consume too many acid generating foods for too long so that our bodies become acidic, it provides an ideal environment in which cancer can flourish. As we explained in Step 1, acidic conditions help maintain the acid envelope around cancer which in turn helps it to invade other tissues and to metastasise. Therefore by using diet to alkalise our bodies we can help prevent cancer and stop it spreading. The recent findings by Japanese scientists, that mature cells may be forced to acquire stem-ness by being shocked in acid[48] suggests another reason why it may be beneficial to adopt an alkali-generating diet.

What to eat to balance your diet

So which foods should we focus on to maintain the body's natural alkalinity? Although most people automatically assume that citrus foods will be acid generating because they contain acid, they actually have quite the reverse effect. When a lemon or other piece of citrus fruit is metabolised in the body, alkalis such as potassium are released.[49]

To maintain the optimum balance we suggest a diet of 60 per cent alkali-generating food to 40 per cent acid generating food to prevent cancer, and a ratio of 80 per cent alkali-generating food to 20 per cent acid generating food to treat cancer.

Acid generating foods:

- All animal protein, including eggs, meat, fish and dairy, is strongly or very strongly acid producing or acid generating. Cheese is the most acid generating food of all, with hard cheese generating up to three times more acidity than roast beef.
- Many cereals and pulses such as lentils and peas are moderately acid generating. Oats and brown rice are strongly acid generating but have other values in an anti-cancer diet, such as their high fibre content, and can be balanced by eating alkali-generating foods. Whole wheat is much less acid generating than suggested in the 'alternative' literature.
- Fizzy drinks and colas high in phosphorus are acid generating.

Neutral foods:

- Most fats and oils are close to neutral.

Alkali-generating foods:
- Most fruit and vegetables, even tomatoes and citrus fruits such as lemons, are alkali generating.
- Herbs and spices, such as ginger and garlic, and dried herbs, such as parsley and coriander, are strongly alkali-generating.
- Drinks low in phosphorus, such as spirits, wine and beer are neutral to alkali generating. Tea, including many herbal teas, many mineral waters and soya milk, are moderately alkali generating or nearly neutral.

You will find a full list of foods which are alkali generating and those which are acid generating in Table A in the Appendix.

Understanding the pH scale

Scientists use a scale based on pH values from 1 to 14 to show how acid or alkaline a solution is. A pH of 7 is neutral, which means there is a perfect balance of hydrogen and hydroxide ions (as in pure water, for example). Values less than 7 are acid, while values greater than this, up to 14, are alkaline. The scale is logarithmic – in other words every increase or decrease of 1.0 in the pH value means that the number of excess hydrogen or hydroxide ions increases or decreases 10-fold. This means that a pH of 6, for example, is 10 times more acid than one of 7, while a value of 5 is a hundred times more acid than one of 7. The same applies on the alkaline scale.

Food Factor 5: Eat vegetable not animal protein

A certain amount of protein is essential for good health – the amino acids contained in protein foods are the building blocks that make up your cells and body tissues and help repair them when they are damaged. But there is now substantial evidence from a range of studies[50] that too much protein – particularly animal protein – is at best unhelpful and at worst dangerous to those at risk of cancer, whereas a plant-based diet is protective.

Why avoid animal protein?

One problem is that animal protein is often high in messenger molecules such as growth factors and hormones that are chemically identical to our own. Oestrogen is a perfect example. We saw in Step 1 how oestrogen, now considered a Category 1 carcinogen by the International Agency for Research on Cancer, can promote breast and ovarian cancers. All vertebrate animals produce oestrogens which can be detected in their produce – meat, eggs and dairy foods – and which end up in the environment in streams

If you used to do this...	Now do this...
Eat a 'full English' with eggs, sausages and bacon	Have beans on toast, bubble and squeak (cooked potatoes and Brussels sprouts/cabbage gently fried in olive oil, or mushrooms on toast. Gently fry some garlic in olive oil, add your favourite mushrooms and cook slowly. Pour some of the oil onto wholegrain or rye toast, add the mushrooms and serve sprinkled with parsley.
Eat lots of processed meat in sandwiches or salads	Eat miso (which has a meaty taste) or dairy-free guacamole in wholegrain sandwiches or with salad vegetables.
Eat meaty soups	Eat vegetable or miso soups instead.
Love the cheese course	Add a course with your favourite vegetables, e.g. steamed asparagus or artichoke hearts with an olive oil, cider vinegar, Dijon mustard and garlic dressing or try sliced raw fennel with lemon juice, olive oil and capers.
Eat lots of meaty burgers	Switch to dairy-free veggie burgers.
Enjoy mince and tatties and spaghetti bolognese	Use quorn or other good meat substitute and make your sauce even more delicious with extra onions, vegetables and lots of tomato paste.

and sea water, in soil, sewage and manure and even in drinking water as a result of excretion.[51]

There is much evidence from studies in the USA, China and Japan that consuming an animal-based diet increases circulating levels of oestrogen, while levels are lower in people on a plant-based diet.[52] Moreover, work published in 2009 showed that American beef (which is treated with hormones) contains much higher levels of oestrogens than Japanese beef.[53]

Oestrogen

Oestrogen is a Category 1 carcinogen and the way in which it promotes cancer such as breast and ovarian cancer was discussed at Step 1. Steroid oestrogens are produced by all vertebrate animals and, as such, they can be detected in produce such as meat, eggs and dairy foods. Their excretion is a major pathway of these substances into the environment. (For full details see Table B in the Appendix.)

Why avoid dairy?

Despite research linking eggs and meat to different types of cancer, the animal protein considered most risky for cancer patients is casein, the main protein found in cow's milk and dairy products (such as yoghurt, butter and cheese). In fact Professor Campbell has argued that casein fulfils all the criteria established by IARC to be a Category 1 carcinogen.[54]

While all this might appear counter-intuitive to those of us brought up with the school milk project and the message that cow's milk is good for us[55] the reality is that it is good for calves, not people. This is still controversial for some oncologists but many eminent scientists, including biochemists, and many research-active doctors are convinced by the evidence.

As recently as 26 January 2012, Harvard University's School of Public Health issued a statement that Dairy is NOT Part of a Healthy Diet (their capitals). The Harvard School of Public

Health declared that the university's new Healthy Eating guide is 'based on the latest science ... unaffected by businesses and organisations with a stake in their messages'.[56] Harvard's 'Healthy Eating Plate', designed for healthy people, not cancer patients, contains minimal dairy based on their scientists' assessment that 'a high intake can increase the risk of prostate cancer and possibly ovarian cancer'.

Professor Colin Campbell's 2006 book *The China Study*[57] contains a wealth of experimental and epidemiological evidence for the association of dairy foods with many types of cancer.

One of the reasons we consider dairy foods to be so dangerous is that they contain a cocktail of highly biochemically active substances, especially hormones and growth factors which are increasingly strongly linked to cancer. Cow's milk has been shown to contain 35 different hormones and 11 growth factors, and one recent study identified 20 pharmacologically active substances in cow's and goat's milk which included many pharmaceutical residues as well as oestrogens.[58]

Twelve years ago, Jane highlighted the problem of the growth factor IGF-1 found in milk, cheese and all milk products. At the time there were relatively few scientific publications on the subject but in the intervening years there has been a wealth of other research confirming her analysis. A high level of circulating IGF-1 is strongly linked to the development of many cancers, and some experts suggest that IGF-1 is to cancer what cholesterol is to heart disease.[59] Jeff Holly, Professor of Clinical Science at Bristol University and a world authority on growth factors, has said, 'The association between IGF-1 and cancer incidence complies with many accepted criteria for causality. There is strong evidence that circulating IGF-1 depends on nutrition.'[60] And the distinguished Harvard University epidemiologist Dr June Chan showed that men with the highest levels of IGF-1 have a 4.3-fold increased risk of prostate cancer compared with those with the lowest IGF-1 levels.[61]

IGF-1 levels have been shown to be significantly higher, and its protective binding proteins (which help to modulate the action of IGF-1) significantly lower, in people eating a Western omnivorous diet *and* in vegetarians who eat eggs and dairy products than in people eating a vegan diet.[62] Scientists at Oxford University's Cancer Epidemiology Unit found that the average blood serum level of IGF-1 was 9 per cent lower in vegan men than in meat-eaters and vegetarians.[63] Other research found that the average IGF-1 concentration was 13 per cent lower and the concentrations of binding proteins were 20–40 per cent higher in vegan women than in meat-eaters and vegetarians.[64] This means that a vegan diet is lower in cancer-promoting molecules and higher in the binding proteins that reduce the action of these molecules.

As we saw in Step 1, Vascular Endothelial Growth Factor (VEGF) is a particularly dangerous growth factor that is strongly implicated in the spread of cancer and, as such, a target for cancer drugs. But as we also learned, VEGF also has a vital role in fighting infection by making tissue more permeable, enabling the movement of white blood cells and driving the body's inflammatory response. It is important in fighting disease in the udders of cows with mastitis and it is estimated from farm records that, at any one time, the mean incidence of mastitis in English and Welsh dairy herds is 47 cases per 100 cows per year.[65] There are increasing numbers of papers in the scientific literature about VEGF in milk, particularly from cows affected by the sort of bacteria that infect the highest-yielding cattle breeds typical of modern industrialised dairy units.[66]

It seems to be assumed that it is our own bodies that produce the excess VEGF levels seen in cancer patients. As yet, there are no studies of the relationship between diet and circulating levels of VEGF as there have been of IGF-1 and diet, but it seems likely that a similar relationship will be found. More research on links between diet and circulating levels of VEGF comparable to that carried out for IGF-1 is needed urgently.

Many of you will be familiar with the emotional debates about funding expensive drugs which may extend the lives of cancer patients by a few months. Many of these drugs are aimed at blocking VEGF. It seems likely, however, that, if a cancer patient is consuming dairy products, they are also consuming VEGF, especially if the milk originated from cows with mastitis. That is not helping them to defeat their illness – and it may be making things worse. It is just one extra reason to avoid milk and other dairy products.

Getting the protein your body needs

If you are going to cut animal protein out of your diet where do you get your protein and what about sources of calcium? It is the first question that most people ask if you say that you are on a vegan diet. There is a widespread view that while animal protein is first-class protein, plant protein is a poor second best. This is not the case – if you combine the right types of vegetable proteins it is every bit as good as eating animal protein and there are plenty of calcium sources other than milk and dairy products.

If you used to do this...	Now do this...
Have lots of dairy milk/yoghurt and sugar with your cereal	Make organic porridge with water, add some oat or soya milk, sprinkle with cinnamon and add molasses and chopped banana.
Put lashings of butter/margarine containing dairy on your toast	Have organic soya spread, hummus, organic peanut or seed butter (make your own by blending sesame, pumpkin or flax seeds in a good-quality blender with olive or sesame oil and a little freshly squeezed lemon juice with sea salt and black pepper to taste) or follow the Spanish and put olive oil on your toast!
Sip milky tea or lattes through the day	Drink green tea with a slice of lemon or lime and herbal teas such as peppermint or fennel.

Have a cheese and pickle sandwich or a cheese salad for lunch	Try hummus and pickle or hummus and sundried tomatoes in wholemeal bread sandwiches or babaganoush instead of cheese with your salad.
Have a dairy fruit yoghurt for lunch	Eat a soya or coconut yoghurt and add extra fruit until you get used to the different taste.
Eat cream of vegetable soups	Make your soups 'creamy' by adding potato. Gently fry a medium brown onion in extra virgin olive oil and when it is soft add crushed garlic and a chopped red or green chilli to taste. Add a good-quality stock made with vegetable stock cubes and a sliced potato. Bring to the boil and simmer until the potato is soft. If you are making soup with hard vegetables such as carrots add them at this stage. Soft vegetables such as leeks or watercress can be added, chopped shortly before serving. Blend and serve in pretty dishes, sprinkled with parsley.
Eat cheesy pizza	Have a Margarita without cheese but add more of your favourite vegetables such as artichokes, peppers or mushrooms.
Love cauliflower cheese	Hummus is a delicious substitute for cheese. Buy organic hummus or make your own by blending a tin of chickpeas with freshly squeezed lemon juice, two tablespoons of tahini paste, a tablespoon of olive oil with black pepper to taste and a little sea salt.
Eat lashings of ice cream and cream	Try some of the delicious soya or coconut ice creams and creams instead or try sorbets and water ices.
Have hot chocolate or cocoa made with dairy milk before bed	Experiment with organic veggie milks instead and add a little extra-dark chocolate or cocoa until you get used to the new taste.

Most edible plant foods provide adequate amounts of protein. Cereals (e.g. barley, oats, rye and wheat), pulses (e.g. peas, beans and lentils), and nuts and seeds all contain protein; and quinoa has a complete range of protein. To ensure you are getting the complete range of amino acids, eat complementary vegetable proteins in the same meal. Nuts, seeds and grains are generally high in tryptophan and sulphur-containing animo acids but low in a type called lysine. However, legumes – beans and peas – are usually high in lysine but low in tryptophan and sulphur-containing animo acids. So combining legumes with nuts or seeds or grain will provide you with the complete protein you need. Here are a few suggested combinations.

- Bean soup with sesame-seed crackers
- Snack mix of raisins, peanuts and sunflower seeds
- Baked beans and brown bread
- Red beans and rice
- Split pea soup with corn bread

What about soya?

Soya also provides a complete range of protein and you can eat it in many forms, as soya milk, traditional beancurd or tofu, tempeh or miso. We do not recommend foods based on concentrated soya protein such as those made to mimic cheese, bacon or other meats. Like other concentrated proteins, these can acidify the body and may also contain unhealthy chemical additives.

Is soya safe?

Concerns have been raised that soya causes breast and prostate cancer or feminises males. That does not even pass the common-sense test. The Chinese, Japanese and other East Asian people have been eating soya in one or more of its traditional forms for at least 3,000 years.[67] In China, where soya has been venerated as one of five sacred foods for at least 2,000 years, there has not been any observable problem from the phyto-oestrogens it contains.[68] There is no problem with lack of male potency or reproductive capacity there or in any other oriental country, and they have one of the lowest rates of hormone-related cancer in the world – or they did until they began to adopt a Western diet. When Jane first visited China she was intrigued to discover that they gave their schoolchildren soya rather than dairy milk in their morning break.

One of the arguments used against soya is that it contains phyto(plant)-oestrogens. We think that the confusion is because of the oestrogen in the name and we explained why they are far less dangerous than animal oestrogens, as mentioned in Step 1.

The three major groups of phyto-oestrogens are:[69]

- Isoflavones, which are particularly common in Eastern diets (for example in soya).
- Lignans, found in high concentrations in grains, seeds such as linseed, and other fibre-rich foods including broccoli and cauliflower. They are probably the most common phyto-oestrogens in the Western diet.
- Coumestans, including coumestrol, one of the more oestrogenic phyto-oestrogens, which are found in various beans, such as split peas, pinto beans, and lima beans, and also in alfalfa and clover sprouts.

Other phyto-oestrogens are found in hops and beer,[70] liquorice[71] and coffee.[72] In fact, they are found in most foods that contain plant material, and human exposure is substantial. Myco-oestrogens are similar molecules produced naturally by fungi, such as the *Fusarium* species, which grows on cereals including corn, barley, wheat, hay and oats.[73]

Like human oestrogens, phyto-oestrogens and myco-oestrogens bind to oestrogen receptors in the body, but they are far weaker[74] and rather than increasing cancer risk, may actually be protective. Isoflavones have been shown to lower the risk of prostate cancer[75] and one of the most recent studies suggests that soya does not increase the risk of recurrence of breast cancer.[76] Another recent study showed that phytochemicals in soya and other legumes protect against endometrial cancer in post-menopausal women.[77] In our bodies they appear to work in a similar manner to the pharmaceutical drugs called *selective oestrogen receptor modulators* (SERMs) and help protect against cancers such as breast cancer.

Nevertheless, we recommend against taking phyto-oestrogens as extracts. Eat the whole food.

You can find out the facts about soya researched by biochemist Justine Butler on the Viva! website.[78]

Best sources of calcium

Calcium is vital for healthy teeth and bones and also helps the heart, nerves, muscles and other body systems work properly, and there are plenty of excellent sources of calcium other than dairy products. The experts at Harvard highlighted the high levels of saturated fat in most dairy products and suggested that bok choy, fortified soya milk, and baked beans are safer choices than dairy for obtaining calcium. In fact, most vegetables are good sources of calcium. Even good orange juice contains more calcium than human breast milk.

Other advantages of a plant-based diet

Of course a plant-based diet has many other benefits – unlike animal foods, unrefined plant foods are high in fibre, which protects against many cancers, especially colorectal and breast cancer.[79] It has been suggested that vegetable proteins reduce cancer risk by helping to balance glucagon and insulin activity, thereby lowering blood serum lipid levels, promoting weight loss and decreasing circulating IGF-1 activity.[80] Plants have also been shown to contain a wide range of chemicals which are cancer protective (see Table C in the Appendix).

Food Factor 6: Get your fats right

Fats are vital for good health, but only in the quantities and forms our bodies have evolved to use. As well as providing a source of energy, fat, like protein, fulfils important structural functions within the body. Your brain, for example, is about 60 per cent fat, and the peripheral nervous system is covered by a fatty substance called myelin which insulates nerves, in the same way that rubber or plastic insulates electric cables. Fat also provides a cushion for delicate organs such as the kidneys and it is present in healthy human breasts. It is found in all of our cells and enables our bodies to absorb the vital fat-soluble vitamins, A, D, E and K. Of course fat is also highly calorific containing more than twice as many calories per gram than either protein or carbohydrates (9 kcal/g as opposed to 4 kcal/g). And although fat provides an important energy store, excess fat, especially fat stored in or around the heart, arteries or liver, can cause serious health problems.

Bad fats

For decades we have been advised to minimise our intake of animal fat, the saturated fat found in butter, cheese, cream, meat and eggs that has been linked to many types of cancer and heart disease. More recently there have been concerns about trans-fatty acids, made by hydrogenating vegetable oil to make margarines and spreads which are similar in structure and behaviour to saturated fats. If you have been diagnosed with cancer you should eliminate saturated and trans-fats from your diet as soon as possible and replace them with some of the healthy, tasty alternatives in the table overleaf. Check the labels on products to make sure they contain no trans-fats.

Substitute good fats for bad

Instead of saturated and transfats focus on mono-unsaturated and poly-unsaturated fats. The latter include most vegetable oils, which are generally liquid at room temperature. Buy oils which are unrefined and cold pressed and store them in dark bottles away from strong light.

Clearly we do not recommend cooking with animal fats such as butter or lard which are high in saturated fat and may contain steroid hormones such as oestrogen which are fat soluble. Many poly-unsaturated oils, such as unrefined sunflower, safflower and flaxseed oil, are unstable at quite low cooking temperatures.

Dietary sources of fats

Saturated fats: eliminate** or reduce*	Trans-fatty acids (TFAs): eliminate**	Mono-unsaturated fats: 'good fats'	Poly-unsaturated fats: 'good fats'
Butter** Cheese** Margarine** Milk** Coconut oil* Fatty poultry* (duck, etc) Palm oil* Red meats*	Most bought cakes** Cooking fats** Margarine** Highly processed foods (commercial mayonnaise, dressings, creams, etc)**	Almonds Cashew nuts Fish Peanuts Pecan nuts Olives and olive oil Walnut	Omega-3s • Cold-water fish and fish-liver oils • Krill oil • Pecan nuts • Pine nuts • Wheat germ oil • Marine algae Omega-6s • Corn oil • Flax oil • Primrose oil • Safflower seeds and oil • Sesame seeds and oil • Soya oil and beans • Sunflower seed oil • Vegetable oil

We also avoid rapeseed and canola oil which, although they are mono-unsaturated, can be goitrogenic[81] – they damage the ability of the thyroid gland in the neck to take up iodine, which can result in enlargement of the gland, a condition called goitre. We recommend cooking with high-quality extra-virgin olive oil (the basis of healthy Mediterranean cooking) or coconut oil (the basis of healthy Thai cooking). Even so it is important not to let the oils over heat – even if you are cooking a stir fry you do not need the oil to start smoking. Poly-unsaturated oils such as sesame oil are less stable when heated but can be added to stir fries after cooking to give extra flavour.

Balance fatty acids

Essential fatty acids (EFAs) are fats that our bodies need to function properly but which we can obtain only from food because our bodies are unable to synthesise them. There are two classes of EFA – omega-6 (linoleic) and omega-3 (alpha-linolenic). Humans are thought to have evolved on a diet with an approximately 1:1 ratio of omega-6 to omega-3 EFAs (see the box below for omega-6 and omega-3 foods), but the ratio in Western diets is now about 15:1 and in some American diets may be as high as 30:1. This high level of omega-6 EFAs is thought to promote inflammation,

Sources of omega-6 and omega-3

Omega-6: Sources of omega-6 fatty acids include pistachios, olive oil, and olives. Gamma linoleic acid (GLA), which some studies suggest helps reduce inflammation, is found in several vegetable oils, including evening primrose oil (EPO), borage and blackcurrant-seed oil.

Omega-3: Good sources of omega-3 fatty acids are flax seeds, pumpkin seeds, sesame seeds, pine nuts, pecan nuts, leafy greens, cruciferous vegetables, walnuts, wheatgerm, soya oil and spirulina. The three main omega-3s that we get from food are alpha-linolenic acid (ALA), eicosapentaenoic acid (EPA) and docosahexaenoic acid (DHA). Our bodies can convert ALA from flax seeds, pumpkin seeds and sesame seeds to EPA and DHA. There are also useful amounts of EPA and DHA in leafy greens, cruciferous vegetables, walnuts, spirulina, wheat germ and soya oil. Fish are usually considered to be the main source of omega-3 fatty acids in our diet, but fish obtain their omega-3s from the marine algae and seaweed they consume and these are also good sources for humans. Hemp seeds, sunflower seeds and grape seeds also have the right balance of omega-6 and omega-3 fatty acids.

predisposing us to cancer, whereas higher levels of omega-3 (a low omega-6:omega-3 ratio) are thought to be protective.[82]

The ratios have become unbalanced because of our heavy consumption of grain-fed meats such as beef, pork and poultry, and our use of refined cooking oils such as soya, corn and sunflower oil, which are all high in omega-6, and are often used in fast-food restaurants, processed food and home cooking. As a cancer patient or someone wishing to avoid cancer, try to eliminate refined omega-6 oils and processed foods from your diet as much as possible, and always read ingredient labels.

Food Factor 7: Good carbs, bad carbs

Carbohydrates should be your body's main energy source – equivalent to the gas and electricity in your home. This food group includes bread, pasta, rice, potatoes, noodles, chapatti, cereals and other starchy foods (complex carbohydrates) as well as fruit and vegetables which also contain sugars (simple carbohydrates). There is probably more confusion over carbohydrates in relation to cancer than any other food group. A few doctors and many therapists even advise patients to cut out fresh fruit because, they say, the sugar it contains will feed cancer. That is frankly ridiculous – all fruit and most vegetables contain some sugars and are internationally recognised as being protective against cancer and other conditions such as heart disease and stroke.

The idea that sugar feeds cancer originates from the work of Otto Warburg. In 1924, Warburg hypothesised that cancer cells generate energy mainly by fermentation or anaerobic respiration, as opposed to healthy cells which generate energy mainly by aerobic respiration – combining glucose with oxygen to produce carbon dioxide, water and energy. Warburg stated that 'cancer, above all other diseases, has countless secondary causes. But, even for cancer, there is only one prime cause. Summarised in a few words the prime cause of cancer is the replacement of the respiration of oxygen in normal body cells by a fermentation of sugar'.[83]

The concept that cancer cells switch to fermentation instead of aerobic respiration has become widely accepted (see Step 1), although it is no longer seen as the *cause* of cancer. However, Warburg's breakthrough has been misinterpreted by some people

Understanding Glycaemic Index

Several anti-cancer diets recommend that you eat all low-glycaemic index (GI) carbohydrates. GI is a way of ranking carbohydrate foods from 0 to 100 based on how quickly they increase blood-sugar levels. High GI foods, like sugar or white bread, are broken down rapidly and raise blood sugar quickly, while low-GI foods, like oats or beans, are digested slowly and release sugar gradually into the blood stream. However, simply relying on GI can be misleading because the impact that a particular food has on your blood sugar levels depends on the amount of carbohydrate it contains, as well as its GI. Glycaemic load (GL), which takes into account the amount of carbohydrate a food contains, is now considered more important than GI in measuring the impact on blood-sugar levels. The texture and type of cooking also affects a food's GL and as foods are often consumed as part of a meal or snack, it is difficult to use the GL of individual foods.

Although it may seem complicated, the take-home message is to eat foods with low-GL values, such as oats, beans and pulses which are rich in soluble fibre, more frequently than those with high values such as cornflakes, bagels and baguettes. The bottom line is that you cannot go wrong if you focus on unrefined, high-fibre, whole-grain cereals and bread, and use raw cane sugar (molasses) instead of rapidly absorbed refined sugary foods and drinks, and refined white bread and cereals. This is the best way to avoid rapid increases in blood sugar and the rapid release of insulin.

as suggesting that if we remove sugars from our diet – even the fructose in fruit – we will starve cancer.

This is simplistic nonsense. All sugars are converted into glucose, which is vital for energy generation. The process takes place in every cell in our body all day, every day. The brain uses glucose as its main fuel and would rapidly shut down without it. If we do not have enough glucose, the body will convert starch into glucose and if that runs out it will convert fats and even proteins. This can lead in some cases to cachexia, or wasting syndrome, involving loss of weight, muscle atrophy, fatigue and weakness. Forcing the body to break down fats and protein is, after all, the basis of the low-carb diets for weight loss. So while we recommend strongly that everyone, and particularly cancer patients, avoids refined white sugar or foods and drinks in which it is an ingredient, we do recommend masses of fruit and vegetables.

Choose unrefined grains

As well as triggering insulin rushes, refined grains such as white rice, white bread, flour and white pasta have been stripped of vital nutrients. In wholegrain foods such as oats, wholegrain bread and rice and rye bread, the bran, germ and endosperm are all still present. The bran is an excellent source of fibre; the germ is a source of protein, vitamins and minerals; and the endosperm supplies carbohydrates, mainly in the form of starch. They are also rich in phytochemicals and antioxidants, which help to protect against some cancers (and diabetes).

The power of fruit and vegetables

Fresh fruit and vegetables are now so widely accepted as being cancer protective by organisations such as the World Health Organisation (WHO) and the National Health Service (NHS) that many governments recommend that we have at least five portions a day. (The Japanese government suggests nine portions a day.) Table C in the Appendix indicates just some of the substances in fruit and vegetables that contain anti-cancer agents. Eat lots of veggies as salads, soups or lightly steamed or stir fried. Some vegetables, such as cruciferous vegetables, contain goitrogens, however, and they should not be consumed raw or as juices. Try to add sea vegetables such as Wakame or Dulse to juices or to soups (after they have been removed from the heat). These are an excellent source of minerals such as iodine, lithium and magnesium. Eat lots of fruit; raw, juiced and lightly poached or as sorbets. Think of the rainbow rule: have as many different coloured fruits and vegetables as possible each day.[84]

Potatoes have had a bad press but organic potatoes eaten with their skins provide starch for energy, are an excellent source of potassium, vitamin C, vitamin B6 and fibre, and contain the anti-cancer substance quercetin. They also alkalise the body more than grain-based sources of starch and contain similar levels of phenolic antioxidants to cruciferous vegetables such as broccoli. Some people also advise against eating tomatoes and red peppers because they belong to the deadly nightshade family. This is nonsense and there are many papers in the peer-reviewed scientific literature about the health benefits of these foods, which contain powerful anti-cancer chemicals such as lycopene.

Food Factor 8: Cut down on salt and sweeteners

While most of us enjoy a sweet treat now and again, we strongly recommend against eating any refined sugars. The distinguished physiologist Professor John Yudkin has described refined sugar as 'pure white and deadly',[85] so avoid it in all its forms including treacle, in jam, chocolate or other products. Strictly, honey is non-vegan and may be eliminated from your diet if you wish to eat an exclusively plant-based diet.

Artificial sugars are equally worrying. There are now more than 10 synthetic sugars on the market including aspartame, made from wood alcohol, and saccharine, which is made from petroleum. Aspartame is used extensively in diet and low-calorie drinks and foods, chewing gum, yoghurt and products for diabetics. We advise strongly against consuming such products.

If you want to add sweetness, use molasses, raw cane sugar which has not had beneficial minerals such as fluoride (which protects teeth) or chromium (which helps maintain steady blood-sugar levels) refined out. Alternatively use raw maple syrup or unrefined stevia, a herbal sweetener that is available from many wholefood shops.

Salt and sodium

As we saw in Step 1, sodium plays an important role in cancer cells' growth, signalling and metastasis so it makes sense to keep your salt intake as low as possible. Keep your intakes of monosodium glutamate (MSG) (often used to flavour soy sauce and cheap meat in prepared meals), baking soda (bicarbonate of soda) and foods and drinks containing sodium sulphites such as wine as low as possible because, as their names suggest, they are also high in sodium.

Flavourings

Herbs and spices will both make your food taste delicious and alkalise the body. They are packed with antioxidants and essential minerals such as chromium (in black pepper) and iron (in cumin) and also contain powerful anti-cancer chemicals. Chilli peppers contain capsaicin while garlic, ginger and turmeric contain substances with diverse anti-cancer actions. Recently cinnamon has been shown to be powerfully anti-angiogenic – helping to stop the formation of new blood vessels – in laboratory in-vitro studies and in animal experiments. For new blood vessels to form, signalling molecules such as VEGF need to bind to receptors on the surface of the endothelial cells lining the surface of blood vessels – a water-soluble cinnamon extract was shown to inhibit this process.[86]

Herbs are also protective – for example, luteolin found in thyme, parsley, peppermint, rosemary and oregano[87] has anti-cancer properties including anti-angiogenesis. Parsley contains two types of anti-cancer components: volatile oils, *myristicin*, *limonene* and *eugenol*; and *alpha-thujene* and t. including *apiin*, *apigenin* (also in basil), *crisoeriol* and *lut*.

- Volatile oils – particularly myristicin present in small amounts in essential oil of nutmeg and to a lesser extent in parsley and dill – have been shown to inhibit tumour formation in animal studies, particularly in the lungs, and help neutralise particular types of carcinogens (like the *benzopyrenes* in cigarette and charcoal grill smoke).[88]
- Flavonoids in parsley have been shown to prevent free radical damage to cells. Like parsley, mint, thyme, oregano, marjoram and basil also contain apigenin which, according to some authors, is as anti-angiogenic as drugs such as Avastin[89] but without the harmful side effects.

Food Factor 9: What to drink

Clean water

Water straight from the tap is the safest and most obvious choice. Remember that even if you buy bottled water in glass bottles, it is not subject to the same legal limits as tap water. A recent study of European bottled water found that in some cases it contained far more arsenic and nitrate than the UK legal limit for tap water.[90] However, in countries where the quality of water treatment is less reliable it may be better and safer to drink good-quality bottled water.

We filter our tap water through activated charcoal in a simple jug filter and take this water with us in a simple aluminum bottle from a sports or camping outlet. Increasingly, restaurants produce their own filtered water.

Coffee and tea

The evidence for coffee drinking is mixed. On one hand it contains caffeine, which acts as a stimulant, as well as promoting the production of the stress hormones cortisone and adrenaline.[91] Decaffeinated coffee has had most of the caffeine removed, but in some cases this involves the use of harmful chemical solvents such as trichloroethylene. However, coffee consumption has been linked to a reduced risk of oral, oesophageal and pharyngeal cancer,[92] a modest reduction in breast cancer incidence in postmenopausal women, not confirmed in decaffeinated coffee,[93] and a reduction in endometrial cancer in people who drank either caffeinated or decaffeinated coffee.[94] According to one study, coffee protects from liver cancer.[95] Another preliminary study found a correlation between coffee consumption and a lower risk of aggressive prostate cancer.[96] Nevertheless, the IARC has classified coffee as a possible human carcinogen because of possible links to urinary and bladder cancer. It also contains carcinogens such as acrylamide and 3,4 benzopyrene, formed during roasting, and some research links it to pancreatic cancer[97] so on balance we recommend that you avoid coffee.

On the other hand, tea, especially green tea, has been shown in many studies to protect against cancer. It has been known for more than a decade that green tea prevents cancer in experimental animals. According to the US National Cancer Institute, tea contains polyphenol compounds, particularly catechins, which are antioxidants and which some studies suggest have more powerful antioxidant properties than vitamin C. Green tea also contains chemicals which may help protect against cancer by inhibiting enzymes required for cancer growth[98] and block potentially harmful gene activity involved in carcinogenesis caused by tobacco smoke or dioxin.[99] Interestingly, research shows that adding cow's milk to tea removes its health benefits.[100] There are also many good herbal teas such as peppermint and camomile which have beneficial properties such as aiding digestion and having calming effects. Drink water, green tea or herbal teas whenever you feel thirsty.

Alcohol

International health organisations like the World Health Organisation and most cancer charities agree that alcohol is one of the best-established causes of cancer.[101,102] A 2011 UK study estimated that 4 per cent of cancer cases in the UK are caused by alcohol and all of them could be avoided.[103] Cancer Research UK say that alcohol increases the risk of liver, mouth and oesophageal (foodpipe) cancers[104] and that even small amounts of alcohol increase your risk of breast cancer.[105] By contrast a recent study[106] showed that moderate drinkers (3–10g per day of alcohol) with invasive breast cancer had a 33 per cent lower risk of death than non-drinkers, and other research found no definite evidence of any significant link between alcohol drinking and bladder-cancer risk, even at high levels of consumption[107] Similarly, a recent meta-analysis of alcohol drinking and gastric-cancer risk indicated a lack of a link except with heavy drinking.[108]

Interestingly, Campbell and Peto reported that levels of alcohol consumption in China and the US in the 1980s were very similar, despite the big disparity in the rates of breast and prostate cancer. When asked about alcohol, Jane always says she would rather have a glass of organic cider or a single malt whisky with water any day than even a teaspoon of milk!

If you do enjoy a drink, we recommend organic cider or spirits such as a single malt whisky diluted in water, but try to drink in moderation. Wine can contain residues of animal protein such as egg white or cow's milk protein used to 'fine' it or clear it of solids (we used to do this by decanting wine) and it is often high in sodium sulphites. If you drink wine, go for red rather than white as it contains the anti-cancer chemical resveratrol and keep to vegan organic wine.

You can help clear your system and neutralise harmful chemicals such as acetaldehyde at any point after drinking alcohol by drinking organic lemon juice diluted with water or alternatively eating seaweed: it contains cysteine which helps eliminate toxic chemicals left behind.

Food Factor 10: Eat nutritious food rather than supplements

Cancer patients are vulnerable and may take lots of costly supplements recommended by therapists whose main aim appears to be to make money. As we have indicated in Step 4 we strongly support herbal medicine as practised by qualified herbalists but there are many products recommended to cancer patients by private clinics that have no reliable evidence base.

Vitamins

When you live a busy, pressured life and your diet suffers as a result, there can be a tendency to compensate by taking vitamin supplements. This should not be necessary if you follow the diet we have outlined above – it will give you all the vitamins you need with the exception of vitamin D3, for which you need sunshine. There is no evidence that supplements are protective – in fact in many studies they have been shown to worsen outcomes in cancer patients.[109] Two studies carried out in the USA in the 1980s, confirmed by later studies, showed that taking beta carotene supplements worsened outcomes for lung-cancer patients, whereas earlier studies had shown good outcomes in those eating diets high in beta-carotene-rich vegetables such as carrots and broccoli. This suggests, again, that it is the whole natural plant rather than some component that has the benefit. We recommend that you have your vitamin D level checked regularly by your GP.

Minerals

There is concern that soils and hence foods produced by conventional farming are now depleted of minerals such as iodine and selenium.[110] Nevertheless we do not recommend taking mineral supplements as, in some cases, they can be harmful. Copper and iron pills can block the uptake of other minerals and generate free-radical cascades that can damage DNA. Calcium supplements neutralise stomach acid causing problems which range from acid reflux to poor digestion of proteins, and leave us vulnerable to infections such as *Helicobacter pylori* and *Clostridium difficile*. By contrast if you eat vegetables or fruit containing calcium and magnesium, they are released appropriately in the intestines – in the alkaline part of the digestive system. The only supplements we recommend are brewer's yeast as a source of trace minerals and B vitamins, and kelp as a source of iodine, lithium, magnesium and other beneficial minerals as well as spirulina and marine algae. Some people may need to take selenium, but ensure that you never take more than 200 micrograms a day or you may develop symptoms of toxicity. In the case of any other supplements we recommend you first consult a qualified herbalist.

Remember that many of the beneficial vitamins, minerals and phytochemicals in fruit and vegetables work synergistically.[111] As Paul M. Coates, Director of the Office of Dietary Supplements (ODS) at the US National Institutes of Health, says, 'Just because a certain compound in food is beneficial it does not mean that a nutraceutical, with the same compound in it, is … Stick to foods such as flavonoid-rich vegetables and fruits, but do not take high-dose supplements or fortified foods.' The advice is simple. Take green tea, not green-tea extracts, and get your lycopene from cooked ripe tomatoes, not pills.

in a nutshell...

- Diet plays a key role in the development and prevention of many cancers – it is estimated that up to one-third of cancers may be attributable to poor diet.
- Prepare and cook food from scratch and avoid pre-prepared and processed food.
- Eat organically as far as possible to avoid pesticide residues and environmental contaminants which may increase cancer risk.
- Cut down or cut out animal protein (meat, dairy and eggs), which affects our levels and mix of hormones and growth factors,

modifies important enzyme activities, causes inflammation and cell proliferation and creates acid conditions in the body – creating an ideal environment for cancer.[112]

- Stick to a varied plant-based diet which provides fibre, antioxidants and phytochemicals which help protect against cancer, maintain the body's alkalinity and provide phyto-oestrogens to counteract the animal hormones that fuel cancer growth.
- Eat whole unrefined grains which help regulate blood sugar, lower insulin levels and provide cancer-protective fibre and nutrients.
- Focus on eating poly-unsaturated and mono-unsaturated fats, and aim to eat more foods rich in omega-3 fats and fewer of those rich in omega-6 fats.
- Eat more cancer-protective fruit and vegetables and avoid taking vitamin and mineral supplements.
- Avoid refined sugars and cut down on sodium – use raw cane sugar, and herbs and spices which contain chemicals with anti-cancer properties.
- Filter your water, drink tea rather than coffee and keep your alcohol intake to a minimum.

step 6
protect yourself with exercise

Exercise may not be the first thing that comes to mind when you think of cancer prevention and treatment, but there is considerable and growing evidence that exercise may help to protect against cancer and prevent it recurring. According to Cancer Research UK, staying physically active – that means around 30 minutes of moderate exercise, five days a week – could help prevent 3,000 cases of cancer every year.

exercise protects

There is now convincing evidence that regular physical activity is associated with a reduction in the overall risk of cancer and that it has a clear protective effect against bowel and breast cancer. As long ago as 2004, a report by the UK's Chief Medical Officer, published by the Department of Health, found that the most active people had a 40–50 per cent lower risk of bowel cancer than the least active.[1] Similarly, post-menopausal women can cut their breast cancer risk by up to 30 per cent by being active – the more active you are, the lower the risk. Since then, further studies have confirmed the protective effect of exercise against bowel and breast cancers. The US National Cancer Institute (NCI) recently concluded that there is consistent evidence from 27 observational studies that physical activity is associated with reduced death rates from these cancers.[2] The likelihood is that this will apply to other, if not all, cancers. In any case, exercise is good for general health.

The evidence for the protective effect of exercise is now so compelling that the American Cancer Society recommends that everyone should get at least 150 minutes of moderate to intense activity, or 75 minutes of vigorous activity per week in order to protect against cancer.

Staying active can help keep cancer at bay

A growing body of evidence also suggests that patients who are physically active after cancer treatment reduce their risk of recurrence and mortality from some cancers, even if they had not been active prior to their illness. Research has shown this to be the case for several cancers including non-small-cell lung cancer, endometrial cancer, prostate cancer and cancer generally among men.[3] These include older patients.[4]

According to Macmillan Cancer Support, physical activity is important at all stages of cancer treatment and beyond. As well as having anti-cancer effects, regular physical activity can help improve self-esteem, emotional well-being, sexuality, sleep disturbance, social functioning, anxiety and pain – and boost confidence in your body. During treatment, staying active can improve or prevent the decline of physical function. In addition, Macmillan say that it can also help with some of the side effects patients experience during and after cancer treatment, such as fatigue and depression.[5] Far from making you more tired, exercising at the right level can actually increase your energy levels. Moreover, it helps look after your heart and bones, reduces the risk of blood clots and plays an important part in avoiding loss of muscle strength and staying a healthy weight. After you have finished treatment, exercise will help you recover from any physical weakness that you may have experienced. It can be helpful even for people with advanced cancer, and help maintain independence and well-being.

What is the difference between moderate and vigorous exercise?

If you are exercising moderately you will be working hard enough to breathe faster, raise your heart rate and start to sweat. Try the 'talk test' – if you are able to talk but unable to sing you are working moderately. Vigorous exercise means that you are breathing hard and fast and your heart is beating much faster than normal – if you are exercising at this level you will not be able to say more than a few words without pausing for breath. As you would expect, moderate exercise will burn fewer calories than vigorous exercise. Typical examples of moderate exercise are brisk walking (3–3.5 mph), leisurely swimming, badminton, mowing the lawn or slow jogging. Vigorous exercise might include power walking (4.5 mph), squash, running or fast swimming.

If you are unused to exercise take it slowly to start with and gradually build up the time and then the intensity of your exercise.

making exercise work for you

What is clear is that exercise throughout your life protects against cancer. The good news is that it is never too late, even if you have been a couch potato all your life. Start moving as soon as possible and you can still make a real difference to your health. The UK Chief Medical Officer's report recommended that frequent, regular, moderate to vigorous activity provides the best protection.

Exercising with a cancer diagnosis

Until quite recently doctors would advise cancer patients to rest. Today, however, they are more likely to encourage them to stay as active as possible. They may even include exercise recommendations in your personal care plan.

What type of exercise, how much and how vigorous it should be varies from person to person. If you have been diagnosed with cancer it will depend on what type of cancer, what sort of treatment you are having, the stage of your treatment, your energy levels and your general level of fitness before cancer. Try and talk it through with a physiotherapist who will help you to come up with the right exercise plan for you.

Patients and their families often worry, quite understandably, that exercise might be harmful or even dangerous. There is now good research evidence that for all but a small number of people, there is no need for concern as long as you are sensible about the type and amount of exercise you do. For example, anyone with cancer which affects their bones or those with osteoporosis should avoid high-impact exercise like running and jumping. No one is going to recommend that a patient who has recently had surgery for prostate or rectal cancer gets straight onto an exercise bike. You will be given guidance on what to avoid and what is suitable for you.

how to get moving

Everyone is different and will respond differently to treatment so a level of activity that is right for someone else may not work for you. For most people, the best idea is to start with a few short spells of walking – just 5–10 minutes – a couple of times a day and gradually build up. Remember that any exercise is better than none and will benefit your health. Listen to your body and do not attempt too much too soon or you will become more tired.

Getting started can be difficult especially if you are not used to exercise, or you have been unwell and inactive for a while. It can help to look at your week and programme the exercise in – write it in your diary, even if it is just 10 minutes, and tick it off when you have done it so you can keep track of your progress. It often helps to find someone to exercise with or to join an organised class or health walk, such as Walking for Health (WfH) (see below).

The good news is that effective exercise does not need to involve complicated work-outs, expensive gym fees or special equipment. Often the simplest – and cheapest – approach is the best.

Walking is free, you can do it anywhere, anytime and it is one of the most beneficial and sustainable forms of exercise available, especially if you do it in the countryside, a park or garden – known as the 'Green Gym' (or by the sea, in the 'Blue Gym'[7]). If you are not used to exercise it can be hard to get started and then maintain your momentum, but a review of different exercise regimes found that a programme that involves walking, where you do not have to attend a gym or sports centre, is most likely to be sustainable.[8]

The WfH initiative organises walks specifically for people living with or after cancer (as well as for people who just want to get fit). The group walks, which take place in accessible green spaces and cater for different fitness levels, are led by patients rather than health professionals. This also helps to develop a supportive community and double the success rate for the walkers.[9] Walk leaders are given professional training, are insured and nationally accredited. The WfH programme for cancer patients is now managed by Macmillan Cancer Support and The Ramblers. You can find your nearest centre on the WfH website.[10] The Countryside Management Service (CMS) runs similar walks, as do many local authorities.

If for any reason walking is difficult for you, there are plenty of other options. Many doctors can now prescribe gym sessions as part of your treatment. Other aerobic exercises include swimming, jogging or competitive sports like tennis.

If none of this appeals to you, why not take up dancing? There are a huge variety of classes on offer from Jazz, Hip-hop and Flamenco to Ballroom and Latin, Salsa and Swing. It is sociable and fun, classes provide a regular routine and there is plenty of evidence that it is just as beneficial as more traditional exercise regimes. Dancing is especially good for older adults: Latin dancing, in particular, has been shown to increase balance and strength in older people, as well as building confidence and a more positive body image.[11] Music provides an added bonus – one study found that groups exercising to music had greater feelings of positive well-being and lower levels of fatigue straight after exercise than other forms of activity, despite burning a similar number of calories.[12]

Dancing has also been used therapeutically with breast-cancer survivors. One study in the USA showed that a structured Dance and Movement program significantly improved the quality of life in breast-cancer survivors, including an improved body image.[13] Another study of breast-cancer survivors similarly demonstrated that life satisfaction could be increased significantly by a traditional Greek Dance program, also decreasing depressive symptoms.[14]

If you cannot find an exercise programme that works for you, just become more active in everyday life. Even gardening and housework can help to build your fitness and body confidence.

The complementary approach

Eastern forms of exercise such as yoga and Tai Chi are based on the balanced use of the body. Tai Chi, for example, can be particularly helpful for patients who experience problems with dizziness, frailty or peripheral sensory neuropathy.

Tai Chi and Qigong both come from the Chinese medical tradition and promote a sense of well-being and peace. Both use gentle movements, controlled breathing and mental imagery and are intended to balance the Chi (or life energy) of the body. Studies have confirmed both types of exercise can increase strength and flexibility and improve balance and circulation. More information is available from Tai Chi Finder at www.taichifinder.co.uk or the Qigong Association at www.qi.org

Yoga is known as a *whole body* system and involves breathing exercises and static postures (known as asanas) and meditation to create harmony between the body, mind and spirit. Evidence from brain scans has demonstrated the beneficial effects of yoga.[15] Developed in India more than 5,000 years ago, yoga is now widely used in the West. There are many different types. Some are gentle, focusing mostly on breathing and meditation exercises, while others are more vigorous and physically demanding. There is plenty of positive evidence for the health benefits of yoga. One recent study found that cancer patients who followed a four-week yoga course after they had completed their treatment had fewer problems sleeping and felt less fatigued.[16] More information about yoga is available from the British Wheel of Yoga at www.bwy.org.uk.

how exercise protects

Although there is still much that we do not understand about the biological processes that make exercise so beneficial, it is thought that physical activity may modify the levels of hormones and growth factors that are implicated in many cancers.[17] In addition, exercise can regulate energy balance and fat distribution, and promote antioxidant defence and DNA repair.

Exercise can also play an important role in helping to maintain a healthy weight, and assist weight loss if you are overweight. Being overweight or obese increases the risk of several types of cancer, as well as diabetes and heart disease.[18]

The NCI study referred to earlier in this chapter also suggests that exercise may result in beneficial changes in the blood insulin levels, insulin-related pathways, inflammation, and possibly even immunity. It has been shown to increase the activities of disease-fighting T-cells and neutrophils, lower the inflammatory response to bacterial challenge and alter circulating levels of inflammatory cytokines.[19] In particular, regular exercise increases production of interleukin-2, which is currently being investigated as an immunotherapeutic cancer treatment in its own right.[20] Being outdoors also increases levels of Vitamin D, sometimes called the 'guardian of the genome'.

Physical activity may have additional specific effects relating to different types of cancer. For example, some experts have suggested it may reduce exposure to hormones such as oestrogen and testosterone that are implicated in hormone-dependent cancers like some breast, endometrial, prostate and testicular cancer. It may speed up the transit of food through the body, which may mean the intestinal tract is less exposed to cancer-causing agents. Exercise may stimulate changes in the levels of insulin, prostaglandin and bile acids to help prevent cells in the colon from proliferating. Improved lung function resulting from exercise may help to prevent lung cancer by minimising the presence of carginogens in the airways.

There is also much evidence of the benefits of exercise in helping to treat the anxiety and depression that can follow a diagnosis of cancer.[21] These findings should come as no surprise since as humans we are designed to be active. Activity by fighting or fleeing was the way our ancestors burned up the adrenaline and cortisol that were released as a result of sudden threats. In today's world, high levels of these hormones are more likely to reflect chronic stress and strain than a response to physical danger. Exercise remains one of the best ways of burning the stress hormones up and reducing their potential to cause long-term damage.

in a nutshell

- Exercise helps to protect against cancer and can aid recovery in patients. It also has numerous other health benefits including protecting against stroke and heart disease, helping to maintain strong bones and weight control.
- Appropriate exercise is safe and beneficial for all but a small minority of cancer patients. Always talk to your doctor before embarking on an exercise programme.
- Start with a small amount of exercise, programme it into your routine and gradually build up.
- Find an activity you enjoy and can easily fit into your life so that you will carry on with it and have fun.

step 7
be aware of
your environment

Human beings do not exist or develop in isolation and, as we have seen, nor does cancer. Like many other chronic conditions it can have multiple causes. Over the span of a lifetime our genetic make-up interacts with and is affected by a multitude of external factors. It has been estimated that more than two-thirds of cancers are linked with environmental factors.[1] We have already looked at some of them – namely the role of diet and stress in the development of cancer – but there is also growing interest in the impact of carcinogenic substances in the environment on cancer risk.

Most of us think of 'the environment' as the world outside our homes but when we talk about environmental carcinogens we are referring to everything that is external to, but interacts with, our bodies. So that could be anything from exhaust fumes, to the cleaning products you use and even the bags you wrap your sandwiches in. Tobacco smoke has long been recognised as a cause of lung cancer – still one of the commonest cancers in men and women worldwide – and is now also linked to more than a dozen other cancers. There continues to be concern about increased levels of radioactivity, which can damage DNA and cause cancer.

The idea that our living and working environment affects cancer risk is not a new one. Back in 1775, Soot Wart or Chimney sweep's cancer, a carcinoma of the skin of the scrotum caused by exposure to soot, was the first reported occupational cancer*. More recently asbestos, used in ship building, railway engineering and building, has become recognised as an important occupational carcinogen*. There are other situations where occupation can increase cancer risk. For example, airline pilots have a high incidence of cancer, probably due to exposure to cosmic radiation, chemicals used in aircraft, and shift work.[2] Even some recreational activities can be associated with cancer – golf-course superintendents have a high incidence of prostate cancer, almost certainly due to the high level of pesticides used to keep the fairway manicured.[3] The table on pages 172–174, based on information published in 2012, shows the links between occupational exposure to potentially hazardous substances and cancer.

In this Step we will look at some of the potentially harmful substances you are likely to encounter in everyday life and the steps you can take to reduce your exposure – and your cancer risk. Our message is simple. We believe that you cannot rely on the authorities to reduce your exposure to carcinogenic chemicals: you need to take charge of cutting your exposure yourself.

the history

Concerns about chemicals in the environment date back at least to the 1920s, when doctors and scientists such as Sir Robert McCarrison and Sir Albert Howard reported that the Hunza and Sikh communities were essentially cancer-free. They linked the much higher incidence of the disease in the West to the development of chemical-based agriculture.[4] In the first half of the 20th century there was a growing number of early warnings about the hazards and risks of chemicals,[5] but it was the publication in 1962 of Rachel Carson's landmark book *Silent Spring*[6] that catalysed public concern, with its description of the damaging effects of pesticides on birds.

---

* Occupational cancer is outside the scope of this book but the subject is fully treated in a report entitled 'Occupational cancer in Britain' by Lesley Rushton and Gareth Evans with the British Occupational Cancer Burden Study Group.

Although evidence of the links between cancer and environmental factors is accumulating, it is still early days. We live in a constantly changing world and it is not possible to provide a definitive assessment of the risks of exposure to harmful substances, simply because we still do not know enough. Of the estimated 140,000+ chemicals on the market today, only a fraction has been thoroughly evaluated to determine their effects on human health and the environment.[7] In some cases we know about the impact on adults but not on children or the developing foetus. We still have very limited understanding of the effects of mixtures or 'chemical cocktails', although we know that environmental contaminants interact with each other and this may intensify their effects. Some substances may be particularly harmful at critical periods of development – in the developing foetus, in early life or during puberty. It is also likely that an individual's genetic make-up may affect their susceptibility to particular contaminants and in some cases exposure can have intergenerational effects – so that genetic damage is passed down through the generations.[8] What's more, many products, especially perfumes and cosmetics, include unidentified substances because manufacturers can claim that naming those substances would damage their commercial advantage.[9]

The information and guidelines in this chapter are based on the best available research and evidence at the time of writing. The idea that there are tens of thousands of potentially carcinogenic chemicals in our day-to-day environment might, at first glance, seem rather scary. But it is important to remember that the science assessing the risks of environmental substances is still relatively new and in the majority of cases the relationship between a chemical and cancer is not one of simple cause and effect. In a very small number of cases we can say with certainty that a substance causes cancer – tobacco is the one that everyone will be familiar with – but in the majority the picture is far more complicated. A substance may have carcinogenic properties – so it may influence cancer risk – but the risk this poses to each individual varies. The risk that a particular substance presents to any one individual will depend on how hazardous the substance is, the individual's level of exposure, the interaction of the substance with other potential carcinogens, other lifestyle factors such as diet, and the individual's own genetic make-up. Disease will develop only when the combination of risk factors reaches a critical point, which tips the body over into cancer. We are well aware that life can never be risk free and the purpose of this chapter is to make you aware of potential hazards and empower you to make changes to your lifestyle and buying habits that can help protect you and your family now and in the future.

What are the authorities doing about the problem?

The International Agency for Research on Cancer (IARC) publishes a list of known and possible carcinogens (see table below) based on an evaluation of the existing human and experimental animal data as well as information on the biological plausibility of carcinogenicity.

Classification of carcinogens by IARC

Group	Risk	Agents
Group 1	Carcinogenic to humans	107
Group 2A	Probably carcinogenic to humans	63
Group 2B	Possibly carcinogenic to humans	271
Group 3	Not classifiable as to its carcinogenicity to humans	509
Group 4	Probably not carcinogenic to humans	1

Group 1 carcinogens include toxic trace elements such as arsenic, cadmium and chromium, which occur naturally and in manmade compounds. In addition, there are natural and manmade radioactive substances, natural and synthetic hormones such as oestrogen, and natural particulates such as asbestos, as well as industrial chemicals like benzene and vinyl chloride. Similar products are found in Group 2, while the Group 3 list – by far the largest – consists of substances that we do not know enough about to be able to classify them.

In the USA the 2008–2009 Annual Report of the President's Cancer Panel 'Reducing Environmental Cancer Risk'[10] includes a great deal of advice on what individuals can do to reduce their exposure.

A recent report from The European Environment Agency (EEA)[11] warned that common chemicals found in household products as well as in pesticides, cosmetics and medicines may be causing a range of medical problems, including cancer. Many are endocrine-disrupting chemicals (EDCs), known to damage wildlife, and there is increasing evidence that they are also harmful to humans, affecting the reproductive system, metabolism, growth and mood. They do this by interfering with our hormones, including thyroid and sex hormones such as thyroxin, oestrogen and testosterone.[12] EDCs can affect any aspect of hormonal synthesis or function, from gene expression to the transport and actions of hormones themselves.[13] EDCs can persist in the environment and have an effect even at very low levels and, worryingly, their effects are not always identified in standard toxicology tests.[14]

There is growing evidence that exposure to EDCs promotes hormone-dependent cancer.[15] It has been linked to testicular cancer[16] and prostate cancer[17] in men and vaginal cancer[18] and breast cancer in women.[19] The EEA have warned that five classes of EDCs need more scrutiny: phthalates, bisphenol A, PCBs (polychlorinated biphenyls), parabens (used in cosmetics and increasingly found in sunscreen) and certain substances used in contraceptive pills. They stopped short of banning any of these chemicals, although, since 2007, using phthalates in toys and childcare articles has been prohibited. Parents should be aware that plastic toys produced before 2007 are likely to contain phthalates.

In 2003 the UK Royal Commission on Environmental Pollution[20] expressed concern about around 30,000 chemicals used in the European Union which had never been comprehensively tested. Their report focused on chemicals used in products that can gradually find their way into the environment and people's bodies. However, in 2007 REACH (Registration, Evaluation, and Authorisation of Chemicals) legislation was enforced throughout the EU, which required manufacturers and users of chemicals to prove the safety of their product. As a result of this legislation many known carcinogenic chemicals were voluntarily withdrawn from the European market by industry. Some legislation does not affect products made outside the EU, however, and in countries such as China and India safety legislation is poor or nonexistent.

A UK-based study of the occurrence of different cancer types and associated carcinogens for different professions and occupations[21]

Profession / occupation	Associated cancer type(s) (% of cases) [those less than 1% not shown]	Relevant carcinogen(s)	Non-associated cancer type(s) (0 %) ND, not determined
Metal workers	NMSC (62), bladder (20), lung (14), sinonasal (4)	Mineral oils	ND
Mining	Lung (83), NMSC (10), bladder (2), mesothelioma (3), stomach (2)	Asbestos, DEE, solar radiation, silica	Bone, brain, leukaemia, liver, thyroid
Printing and publishing	Lung (98)	Mineral oils, cobalt, radon, solar radiation, tetrachloroethylene	Bladder, brain, cervix

Welders	Lung (97), melanoma-eye (3)	Fumes containing metals (e.g. nickel, cadmium, and chromium VI)	ND
Manufacture of industrial chemicals	Lung (60), mesothelioma (26), larynx (5), NHL (3), stomach (2)	Asbestos, sulphuric acid, TCDD, cobalt, chromium VI, arsenic, radon, inorganic lead, silica	Brain, leukaemia, liver, LH, MM
Painters (not construction)	Lung (66), stomach (18), bladder (16)	Arsenic, cadmium, chromium VI compounds, asbestos, formaldehyde, benzene	ND
Manufacture of pottery, china and earthenware	Lung (63), NMSC (23), NHL (9), STS (31)	Silica, TCDD, solar radiation, radon, cobalt	Cervix, larynx, oesophagus, sinonasal
Electricity, gas and steam	NMSC (62), lung (26), mesothelioma (10), oesophagus (2)	Solar radiation, asbestos, silica, tetrachloroethylene, DEE, radon, arsenic	Bladder, bone, cervix, larynx, leukaemia, liver, sinonasal, stomach, thyroid
Manufacture of other non-metallic mineral products	Lung (88), NHL (6), bladder (3), NMSC (1.5), STS (1.5)	Silica, TCDD, DEE, arsenic, solar radiation	Leukaemia, liver, sinonasal
Manufacture of wood and wood and cork products, except furniture	Lung (78), sinonasal (9), nasopharynx (4), NMSC (3), NHL (3), leukaemia (1.5), STS (1.5)	Arsenic, TCDD, wood dust, cobalt, DEE, radon, solar radiation, formaldehyde	Bladder

Key to table: DEE, diesel-engine exhaust; ETS, environmental tobacco smoke; LH, a type of prostate cancer; MM, multiple myeloma; NHL, non-Hodgkin's lymphoma; NMSC, non-melanoma skin cancer; STS, soft-tissue sarcoma; TCDD, a type of dioxin.

Profession / occupation	Associated cancer type(s) (% of cases) [those less than 1% not shown]	Relevant carcinogen(s)	Non-associated cancer type(s) (0 %) ND, not determined
Manufacture of glass and glass products	Lung (74), NHL (18.5), STS (6), NMSC (1.5)	TCDD, silica, arsenic, cobalt, solar radiation	Bladder, cervix, leukaemia, nasopharynx, oesophagus, sinonasal
Manufacture of paper and paper products	Lung (61), mesothelioma (30), larynx (5), oesophagus (4)	Asbestos, sulphuric acid, TCDD, radon, tetrachloroethylene, cobalt, DEE	Bladder, cervix, leukaemia, LH, sinonasal, stomach, STS
Shift work	Breast (100)	Abnormal light cycle	ND
Personal and household services	Lung (52), oesophagus (19), mesothelioma (10), bladder (5), ovary (5), NHL (4), NMSC (2), cervix (2)	Asbestos, tetrachloroethylene, soots, DEE, ETS, aromatic amines, solar radiation, radon	Liver, nasopharynx
Land transport	Lung (76), mesothelioma (12), bladder (10)	DEE, asbestos, solar radiation, radon, ETS, tetrachloroethylene	Bone, cervix, larynx, liver
Sanitary and similar services	NMSC (76), lung (21), mesothelioma (3)	Solar radiation, asbestos, ETS, DEE, radon	Bladder, bone, leukaemia, liver, stomach, thyroid
Recreational and cultural services	NMSC (81), lung (19)	Solar radiation, ETS, radon	ND
Financing, insurance, real estate and business services	Lung (95), NMSC (5)	ETS, radon, solar radiation	ND

Three potential carcinogens to avoid

All of these harmful man-made chemicals are now ubiquitous in the environment.

Phthalates are commonly used as plasticisers, ensuring that normally brittle plastics remain soft with almost 90 per cent used in PVC, to improve its flexibility and durability.[22] As well as being found in medical devices and food wrappings, they are also used as solvents in many cosmetics such as hairsprays, deodorants, nail polishes and perfumes,[23] and even in time-release pharmaceutical capsules.[24]

The risks: As well as leaching into their surroundings phthalates evaporate and can concentrate in enclosed spaces. The new-car smell and the plastic smell of some indoor tennis and squash courts come from plasticisers. They may affect hormone levels – one study found that men with average amounts of phthalates in their urine had lower levels of testosterone and oestrogen in their blood.[25] Other research suggests that they may be a factor in testicular dysgenesis syndrome which includes a range of conditions from poor sperm quality to, in the worst cases, testicular cancer.[26]

Bisphenol A (BPA) is one of the highest-volume chemicals produced worldwide with an estimated annual production exceeding 8 billion tons, approximately 100 tons of which may be released into the atmosphere.[27] BPA is a chemical used in plastics, especially polycarbonates, which are commonly used to make water bottles, baby's bottles, some plastic cups, and the seams and the linings of cans containing food.

Heat causes the chemical to leach into food, so putting hot food or drinks in plastic containers or using these containers in microwave ovens can increase exposure. Tinned goods have a plastic lining that releases BPA when heated prior to sealing, but fresh, bottled or frozen foods are unlikely to be contaminated. Pottery or metal cups are better than plastic ones, including for travel.[28]

The risks: BPA has been linked to increases in leukaemia and testicular interstitial cell tumours[29] and increased risk of other types of cancer,[30] including breast cancer,[31] prostate cancer[32] and neuroblastoma.[33]

Polychlorinated biphenyls (PCBs) were banned in the US and Europe in the late 1970s but are still present in the environment because of releases from poorly maintained hazardous waste sites, improper dumping of PCB wastes in other landfills and incinerating PCB-containing items.[34] They were previously used extensively in transformers, capacitors and other electrical equipment, in oils for motors and hydraulic systems, adhesives, thermal insulation materials, oil-based paint, dyes, and many other products.

The risks: PCBs are linked to liver and cancers of the bile duct and are suspected carcinogens for breast cancer,[35] prostate cancer,[36] melanoma[37] and non-Hodgkin's lymphoma. IARC classifies PCBs as probably carcinogenic to humans, but recent research by the US National Toxicology Program has confirmed that PCB126 (Technical report 520) and a binary mixture of PCB126 and PSB153 (Technical report 531) are carcinogens.[38]

Becoming aware of the dangers

For the most part we expose ourselves to carcinogens because we inadvertently breathe them in, they are in our food and drink or they find their way into our bodies through our skin or hand-to-mouth touching. Step 5 provides detailed advice on how to avoid potentially harmful chemicals in food and water. In this Step we will help you to identify the danger areas and reduce your exposure.

the big three

By limiting your exposure to the three Ps – pesticides, perfumes and plastics – you can rapidly and dramatically reduce your exposure to carcinogenic chemicals, including EDCs. If you cut down on buying and using products containing the three Ps you will indirectly help yourself and others as this will reduce contamination of the environment by accidental releases during chemical manufacture, spills, poor handling and storage.[39]

Pesticides

At home

Pesticides and herbicides are found in a wide variety of common home and garden products. In fact more than 60 pesticides are approved for non-professional use in the UK[40] as weed and pest killers in the garden, to treat home infestations (of cockroaches or moths for example), to eliminate parasites like fleas in cats and dogs as well as in human and veterinary medicine. We recommend that you employ professionals to treat any infestations at home and ventilate your home well afterwards.

Several pesticides are carcinogens[41] and more than 100 are listed as EDCs[42] by the UK and German environment agencies and WWF.[43] Exposure to certain pesticides, such as the insecticides Dicofol and Tetradifon, has been linked to prostate cancer.[44] The risk of leukaemia increases by four to seven times for children, aged 10 and under, whose parents use home or garden pesticides.[45] The risk of childhood brain cancer is associated with the use of pesticides, such as carbaryl and diazinon, that may be available in garden shops. Even cut flowers may contain significant amounts of pesticide, but levels are not monitored because they are not food – although pesticide-related illness, including higher than normal levels of cancer, has been reported among growers and sellers of flowers.[46] Wash your hands well after handling but ideally stick to pot plants!

Over-the-counter shampoos to treat head lice in children may contain malathion, permenthrin and carbaryl – which are EDCs, and there have been suggestions of a link between these shampoos and childhood leukaemia.[47] Rather than using chemicals on your child's head, invest in a good 'nit comb' and use it to comb tea tree oil through their hair. This is an effective way of removing eggs and lice.

Outside the home

Living in or visiting rural areas can expose you to agricultural pesticides.[48] Studies show that droplets of pesticides applied by tractor can travel up to 60 metres.[49] Pesticides are released from areas where agricultural animals are reared, especially in intensive battery farms or sheds in megadairies. Parks, streets, playing fields and public areas are also kept free of pests and weeds using a variety of pesticides.[50] In the UK large parks have the least pesticide contamination and some, including the royal parks, do not use pesticides at all.

Travel and recreation can all increase your exposure. Pyrethroid insecticides, often combined with other substances to increase their toxicity, are sprayed sometimes in aircraft flying between countries[51] and may be kept circulating by the plane's air-conditioning system. Herbicides, insecticides and rodenticides are routinely used on golf courses, and golf-course superintendents have been shown to have increased mortality from non-Hodgkin's lymphoma and brain and prostate cancer with rates comparable to other pesticide-exposed groups.[52]

Limit your exposure

- Wherever possible, avoid products listed as 'category 1' carcinogens by IARC – you can find a list on the website (http://monographs.iarc.fr).
- If you have to use such products at home do so in well-ventilated areas to avoid inhaling fumes. Open windows and if you use an exhaust fan, make sure the air leaves the building and is not simply being recirculated indoors. Take plenty of fresh-air breaks.
- Use adequate skin, eye, and respirator protection if applying harmful products.
- Read all labels carefully before using products and follow the directions for use as closely as possible. Never use more than the recommended amount.
- Leave products in their original container with the label intact and store in a shed or garage rather than in the house.
- Never put household products in food or drinks containers.
- Do not mix products unless the label directs you to do so. Even different brands of the same product may contain incompatible ingredients.
- If you are pregnant, avoid exposure as much as possible. Many products have not been fully tested for their effects on the unborn.
- Do not eat, drink or smoke while using hazardous products. Traces of hazardous chemicals can be carried from hand to mouth.
- Clean up after using hazardous products. Carefully seal containers. Keep the area well ventilated for several hours after use.
- Practise organic gardening, buy organic food and cook from scratch instead of using ready-made food.

Plastics

Plastics are ubiquitous in our world and hazardous chemicals are involved at all stages of their manufacture, use and disposal.[53] In the first study to look at what happens to the billions of pounds of plastic waste floating in the world's oceans, scientists reported that plastics – thought to be virtually indestructible – decompose quickly, releasing potentially toxic substances such as bisphenol A into the water or into the bodies of animals that have ingested them.[54]

The real danger of many plastic products such as soft and semi-soft toys and bottles made from plasticised PVC or polyurethane, and textiles made from plastic fibres, is that they leach hazardous fat-soluble chemicals into their surroundings. A recent study found that a third of the plastics tested, including 5 out of 13 products intended for children, released residual chemicals, chemical additives and degradation products even when washed with just pure water.[55]

Plasticisers not only leach into their surroundings, they also evaporate and become concentrated in enclosed spaces such as cars and indoor sports courts. Levels have also been reported to be high in children's nurseries, which frequently have lots of plastic toys.[56] Food-contact materials generally are considered an underestimated source of EDC exposure in humans.[57] Plastic water bottles may be problematic – water bottled in the plastic polyethylene terephthalate showed three times the oestrogenic activity of water from the same spring which was in glass bottles.[58]

Limit your exposure
- Buy drinks in glass bottles rather than plastic and use glass bottles to store drinks.
- Avoid plastic food wrap and do not store food in plastic boxes. Use foil or paper instead. This is especially important for children.
- Buy products made in the EU rather than countries which produce cheap but potentially less safe products, especially children's toys.[59]

- Avoid casual chewing of plastic objects such as ballpoint pens!
- Wash hands frequently.
- Cut down on the use of plastics at home – try to use china rather than plastic bowls for example. By cutting down on plastics you will also be helping to protect the environment by reducing the massive amount of non-recyclable plastic waste that is dumped in landfill sites every year.

Perfumes

Perfumes are present in a wide range of personal-care and home products, as well as in perfume itself. Most – even expensive brands – are made from synthetic chemicals, the manufacturers do not have to disclose the ingredients and there is now growing evidence that these concoctions are hazardous. A recent study by The Campaign for Safe Cosmetics and the Environmental Working Group identified hormone-disrupting chemicals and allergens, many of which were not on product labels, in a group of big-name fragrances. The products tested contained an average of 10 chemicals that can cause allergic reactions, including asthma, wheezing, headaches, and contact dermatitis. Some contained 12 different hormone-disrupting chemicals, including some that mimic oestrogen, and are known to be involved in the development of breast cancer.

This is alarming because, unlike food and drugs, cosmetics can be sold without pre-approval[60] under regulations which predate public awareness of the hazards of chronic low-level chemical exposure.[61] European REACH legislation also fails to protect people from hazardous chemicals in perfumes and cosmetics.

What you put on your face and body

In 2012 the US personal care products (PCP) manufacturing industry had a combined annual revenue of about $38 billion.[62] That amounts to an awful lot of chemicals applied to deodorise, protect us from sunburn, supposedly prevent wrinkles or make us look good by applying lipstick or eye make-up. Many of these products are heavily marketed using glamorous airbrushed models and celebrities who promote some new 'breakthrough' ingredient that promises to revolutionise your skin care. Just like the perfume industry, however, many of these products contain EDCs such as phthalates and parabens.[63]

Conventional deodorants and/or cosmetics used by women (and increasingly by men) may contain chemicals, such as parabens, formaldehyde, petrolatum (petroleum), propylene glycol, triclosan, TEA (triethanolamine), DEA (diethanolamine), as well as colouring agents. Also, many PCPs include phthalates such as dibutyl phthalate in nail polish, diethyl phthalate in perfumes and lotions, and dimethyl phthalate in hairspray.[64] These chemicals can build up in the body – for example, parabens from underarm deodorants, sunscreens and other cosmetics was found in all 20 samples of breast-cancer tissue analysed in one study.[65]

Protecting your skin from sun damage is important but chemically based sunscreens are not the answer: many contain parabens[66] and in some the chemical filters they contain generate free radicals, which can make skin age. Some of the ingredients in sunscreens sold in Europe and Asia[67] could not be used in the States as they have not been FDA approved. The most effective way of protecting your skin from the sun is to stay out of it, or cover up. As a geochemist, Jane worked for years in the field, sometimes in hot countries, and always wore a large shady hat and covered up to protect her skin except for a short period of time each day to build up her levels of free vitamin D. Now in her 60s, she still has few wrinkles and is often invited by women's groups to give her talk entitled 'Beauty from the Inside Out!'

EU and US regulations have different approaches to the way that ingredients in PCPs are treated. Any component that goes into a PCP is now covered by the new REACH regulation for chemicals in the EU,[68] which includes hazard and environmental risk assessment. By contrast US law does not presently require the disclosure of chemical ingredients in PCPs.

Limit your exposure

- Try to avoid using highly marketed 'wonder' products and instead use products based on simple chemicals without dyes or perfumes which usually have names indicating that they are ecologically/environmentally friendly.
- Check that the make-up and other products you buy are free from phthalate and parabens. This may not be clear on the ingredients list so you may need to contact the manufacturer.
- There is a growing number of companies, which sell make-up and other personal care products made from plant-sourced ingredients (many of them organic) without the use of undesirable synthetic chemicals. They include Love Lula (www.lovelula.com), Content (www.beingcontent.com) and The Organic Pharmacy (www.theorganicpharmacy.com).
- Go natural. Forget the artificial air fresheners, candles and room sprays. Open the windows instead.
- Make it simple. Use pure simple soap rather than face or body wash and natural products such as gel straight from the Aloe vera plant (but not aloe-vera creams full of preservatives) to moisturise and protect skin from moderate sunlight. You can also use witch hazel to remove grease and act as an astringent and natural salt-stick deodorants (available from health shops).
- Buy fragrance-free personal care and home products wherever possible. You can find out more on the dailygreen website.[69]
- Remember that the condition of your skin depends far more on a good diet, plenty of exercise, avoiding sun damage, not smoking, not taking recreational drugs and going easy on the alcohol. Putting any amount of expensive cream on your face and body will not overcome the damage inflicted by these lifestyle factors.

other danger areas

The hairdresser

Hairdressers use a range of chemicals, from colourants and bleaches, shampoos and hair-styling preparations to nail and skin-care products thought to contain several thousand different chemicals.[70] One of the main hazards is from hair dyes, which can contain several Category 2 or 3 carcinogens.[71] A visit to the hairdresser may also expose you to volatile solvents, propellants and aerosols (from hairsprays), formaldehyde, methacrylates (in nail-care products) and trace quantities of nitrosamines. Many of these chemicals are also in home-use products.

Limit your exposure

Get your hair coloured by a professional hairdresser, who will ensure your exposure is minimised. Avoid hairsprays and use light shades if you can, because in general the darker the dye the more toxic it is likely to be. If you are older, going lighter works better with your changing skin tone. Jane has her hair streaked using peroxide, and then a blonde over-colour is applied and left on for about 10 minutes. All this is done by an expert hairdresser who ensures the chemicals do not touch her scalp. She refuses hairsprays and any other chemicals she considers unnecessary. Mustafa enjoys having grey hair!

Medical and dental care

The main risk here is exposure to ionising radiation, especially from CT scans. Some 1,861 cases, or 0.6 per cent of all cancers diagnosed in the UK in 2010, may have been caused by diagnostic radiation (see Figure 7.1).

In the USA the dose of radiation from medical sources is far higher – it is estimated that it now makes up almost 50 per cent of a person's average annual dose, mainly as a result of the increasing use of hospital CT scans and interventional fluoroscopy. It has been estimated that the number of CT scans in the USA increased from about 3 million in 1980 to 62 million in 2006.[72] The dose from medical interventions is now more than a hundred times the average dose from the nuclear industry (< 0.2 per cent). One CT scan typically delivers a dose 500 to 1,000 times (between 50 and 100 milliSievert/mSv) that of a conventional chest X-ray (0.1 mSv) and 30 to 60 times the dose used in a dental X-ray (1.6 mSv).[73] Data like this have led to a re-evaluation of the risks associated with the use of CT scans in medicine, especially paediatric medicine.

Another concern is exposure to phthalates and bisphenol A from plastics used in medical care, including in tubing and drips and in some pharmaceutical formulations.[74]

Limit your exposure
- If your doctor recommends a scan, discuss it in detail. Outline your concerns about the radiation risks and the estimated number of CT-scan-induced cancers[75] as many are unaware of this. Ask if it might be possible to have an MRI scan or ultrasound instead. CTs (computerised tomography) result in far higher doses of ionising radiation than other forms of investigation, including conventional X-rays.
- Read drug information leaflets carefully and if you are concerned ask your pharmacist to suggest an alternative and ask your doctor to prescribe this. Some of the lurid colours of pills are azo dyes derived from coal tar. Again check with your pharmacist and doctor if you are concerned.
- Many people have their mercury amalgam replaced with white composite fillings, but many of these leak bisphenol A. Ask your dentist to ensure that any white fillings are free of this chemical.

Mobile phones and base masts
There is ongoing debate and intensive research into the potential dangers of mobile phones and base masts. Early studies, generally,

found no link between mobile phone use or proximity to base masts and cancer, but some recent studies have shown varying degrees of association, particularly to forms of brain cancer.[76] In 2011 IARC classified radiofrequency electromagnetic fields as a possible human carcinogen.[77]

Limit your exposure
- Keep a normal landline and use it as much as possible instead of a mobile telephone.
- When using a mobile phone change the ear you are using to listen every few minutes.
- If you are concerned about mobile phone masts in your area, check out your exposure by consulting your nearest branch of the Environment Agency.

at home and away

Many regions of the USA, Europe and the Middle East are affected by high levels of natural radioactivity mainly caused by radon gas, or high levels of arsenic, another Category 1 carcinogen, or both.

Radon
Radon is a radioactive decay product of uranium, which can seep into homes in high-radon areas from the underlying ground and soil gas. It is invisible, odourless and tasteless, but it and its decay products can cause lung cancer by irradiating sensitive cells in lung tissue.[78] The mean radon level in the UK is 20 Bq, slightly less than half that in the USA (46 Bq). The most recent available figures show that the number of lung-cancer deaths in the UK in 2006 attributable to residential radon exposure totalled 1,100.[79] The death toll in the United States is far higher. According to the US Environmental Protection Agency[80] radon-induced lung cancer is the second leading cause of cancer death claiming 21,000 lives every year.

The level of radon and its decay particles in the air increases in stagnant air, such as in mines, caves, or homes without adequate ventilation.[81] Radon levels in the UK vary 100-fold between different parts of the country. The highest levels are found over the granites of southwest England and, to a lesser extent, the

Ionising radiation
One CT scan gives a dose of between 50 and 100 mSv

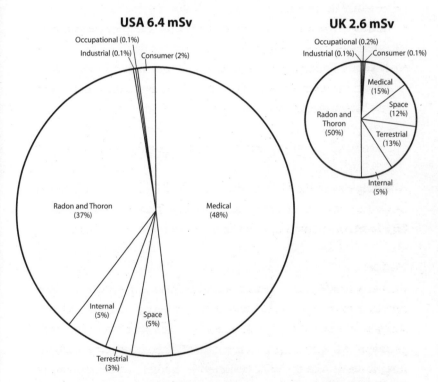

Figure 7.1 *Sources of ionising radiation and their estimated doses as experienced by individuals living in the UK and USA. The overall average dose is 2.6 mSv in the UK but 6.4 mSv in USA (represented by the sizes of the circles). Each section of the circle represents a different radiation source and its size is proportional to the dose. The biggest difference between the two countries is in the extent of the use of radiation for medical purposes.*

Aberdeen granites in Scotland, the limestones of the Derbyshire Peak District and the phosphatic ironstones of Northamptonshire. Figure 7.1 shows that the average annual radiation dose to the UK population from rocks, and radon (and thoron), is approximately 63 per cent of the total radiation dose.[82]

Arsenic

In the UK high arsenic levels often go hand in hand with high radon levels, for example over the mineralised granites in Cornwall. Maps showing the distribution of these substances are available from the British Geological Survey.[83] Arsenic is not just a well-known poison: long-term exposure can also cause skin and bladder cancer. Normal cells can become cancerous when treated with inorganic arsenic[84] and when cancer cells are placed near normal stem cells, these stem cells rapidly acquire the characteristics of cancer stem cells.[85] This may explain why arsenic often causes multiple tumours of many types to form on the skin or inside the body.

The problems of arsenic contamination are widespread. It has been estimated that between 33 and 77 million people in Bangladesh, out of the total population of 125 million, are at risk of arsenic poisoning from drinking naturally arsenic-contaminated groundwater,[86] and chronic arsenic poisoning has also been reported from Argentina, Chile, China, Hungary, India, Mexico, Nepal, Pakistan, Sweden, Taiwan, Thailand and the USA.[87] The problem is caused mainly by naturally high concentrations of arsenic in drinking water, although in China it is as a result of burning arsenic-rich coal.[88]

There may be problems with arsenic contamination closer to home. Chromated copper arsenate (CCA), a wood preservative used since the mid-1930s, is a common source of arsenic in older homes and even play equipment. It can be recognised by the greenish tint it gives timber. Although its domestic use was banned by the European and USA authorities in 2000, rapidly followed by several other countries, some industrial and agricultural uses are still permitted. However, the point of wood preservatives is just that. CCA preserves wood for many years so it may still be found in fencing, decking, sheds and other preserved timbers, including those used in buildings.

Over time, small amounts of arsenic may leach out of the treated timber into surrounding soil, resulting in high concentrations in some cases.[89] There is a more serious risk if CCA-treated timber is burnt in confined spaces such as a domestic fire or barbecue. Although disposal by burning should be performed only in approved incinerators, scrap CCA-treated construction timber continues to be widely burnt through ignorance, in both commercial and domestic fires. Disposal of large quantities of CCA-treated wastes or spent timber at the end of its lifecycle has been traditionally through controlled landfill sites.

Limit your exposure

- Learn if you live in an arsenic- or radon-affected area by referring to maps from the British Geological Survey.
- Anyone concerned about levels of radon in their environment, including home, can consult the Health Protection Agency (HPA) for help and advice.
- If you live in an arsenic-affected area, be careful about eating too many home-grown vegetables. Do not add too much organic matter, such as manure or compost, because this could make the arsenic easier for the plants to absorb.
- If you live in a radon-affected area, ask for the help of the HPA which will determine the levels of radon in your home and advise on how to reduce them.
- Since radon is a heavy gas, try to open windows and doors downstairs at least once a day.

at home

Indoor air quality can be a major concern. According to the UK's Building Research Establishment, poor air quality has a major influence on the health of building occupants. People in Europe spend at least 90 per cent of their time indoors, so that their exposure to many air pollutants is largely indoors. The pollutants include volatile organic chemicals (VOCs), gases such as nitrogen dioxide, ozone and carbon monoxide, particulate matter and fibres, and biological particles such as bacteria, fungi and pollen. Other indoor contaminants come from burning fuels and candles, emissions from building materials, cleaning products, furnishings and electronic equipment (especially brominated flame retardants). New building products can be particularly important sources of pollution. In one survey, nearly 100 volatile organic compounds, of which 10 are regulated in the US as toxic or hazardous chemicals, were found in six samples of fresheners and laundry products.[90]

The impact that pollutants have on health depends on how toxic and concentrated they are and how long people are exposed to them. The effects range from odour to irritation to serious toxic effects. The control of pollutants depends on both tackling their sources and having adequate ventilation with 'fresh' outdoor air. In the USA a five-year study of 600 homes in six cities by the Environmental Protection Agency (EPA)[91] showed that peak concentrations of 20 toxic compounds – some linked to cancer – were 200 to 500 times higher inside some homes than outdoors, reflecting the proliferation of synthetic chemicals in consumer products and furnishings.

Limit your exposure
Use of some potential carcinogens in your home (such as brominated flame retardants in computers and furnishings) cannot be avoided. To minimise your exposure:

- Use cleaning products made from simple, environmentally friendly chemicals.
- Have lots of green plants in your home to clean the air.
- Follow the guidelines on the prevent cancer website.[92]

the problem of waste disposal

In recent years there has been concern over the release of hazardous chemicals from landfill sites and incinerators. Disposal of plastics, for example, causes the release of hazardous chemicals, and poorly operated incinerators can result in the emission of carcinogenic dioxins.

The evidence around landfill sites, including those containing hazardous waste, is conflicting. An initial study in 1999 in Montreal, Quebec, found that men living within 1.25 km of a landfill site had an average two-fold increased risk for pancreatic, liver and kidney cancers and non-Hodgkin's lymphoma.[93] By contrast, two nationwide studies in the UK between 2000 and 2002 showed no increase in cancer in those living near landfill sites.[94] In a study in 2005 in Italy, there was a slight increase in mortality but not the incidence of liver and bladder cancer and non-Hodgkin's lymphoma.[95] More recent studies have found no causal relationship between cancer incidence and living near to landfill sites.[96]

There is more evidence of problems with incinerators. A study in 1997 showed that former workers from a municipal solid-waste incinerator in Italy were at increased risk of gastric cancer,[97] while residents living near incinerators throughout the UK had an increased liver-cancer risk.[98] The risks of childhood cancer, leukaemia, non-Hodgkin's lymphoma and sarcoma have also been shown to be two to three times higher in people living close to incinerators, which has been attributed to increased dioxin exposure.[99] The incidence of non-Hodgkin's lymphoma has also been shown to be increased by high levels of dioxin exposure close to incinerators.[100] Women exposed to high levels of pollutants from incinerators may be more at risk than men according to one recent study.[101]

Limit your exposure

If you are concerned about sources such as landfill sites or incinerators in your area you can check out your exposure by consulting the branch of the Environment Agency nearest to where you live.

in conclusion...

In this chapter we have highlighted the known, most significant cancer-causing substances in the environment. We hope that, armed with this knowledge, you can now make informed choices about what you buy and how you live. Following these simple guidelines will mean that you significantly limit your exposure to harmful substances and protect your health in the process.

- Avoid using chemical pesticides, including insecticides and herbicides, whenever possible and look for environmentally friendly alternatives. If you have to use chemically based products follow the instructions carefully and store them safely, ideally outside your home.
- Read labels on household products carefully and avoid those containing potentially dangerous substances.
- Make a decision to limit the amount of plastic in your home and avoid plastic storage boxes and food wrapping. Ensure that you buy toys and other plastic products made within the EU.
- Choose natural, unperfumed, personal-care products.
- If you are offered a CT or other scan question your doctor about why it is necessary and ask if there is any alternative.
- Knowledge is power and it will help you to make the choices that will help you protect yourself and your family. Keep yourself informed and up to date. See Resources (page 241) for further sources of information.

step 8
manage stress

Being given a diagnosis of cancer is at best shocking, and at its worst truly terrifying for many people. Within seconds, life as you know it is turned upside down and you are thrown into an unfamiliar world of hospital appointments and treatment plans. So when friends and acquaintances then tell you that you must 'think positively' it can feel like the final straw, especially if the cancer diagnosis comes at a time when there have been other significant issues in your life.

Being resolutely positive can be hard when you feel shocked, frightened and uncertain, and however well meaning the advice, it can leave people feeling guilty that they are not making more progress against their cancer.[1] If only they could try harder to banish the negative feelings and think more positively, then they would get better. When the cancer comes hot on the heels of other stressful life events some patients and their families become fearful that even everyday life events – an argument with a loved one, or the car breaking down – will aggravate their cancer.

In this Step we will try to help you to understand more about how stress works, and to find practical ways to identify and manage the stressors in your life and the anxiety and depression that can result from a cancer diagnosis, whether it is a first diagnosis or the news that cancer has returned. While the main thrust of this chapter is aimed at people who have had a cancer diagnosis, the information and advice is equally applicable to anyone who wants to take steps to protect themselves against cancer.

understanding stress and strain

Although health professionals tend to use the term stress for both the *causes* of pressure on an individual – life's problems – and the *effects* that those problems have – your physical and emotional reactions – this can cause confusion. It is much easier to understand the health effects of stress and how we can improve our resilience if we define stress and strain in the more precise way that engineers and scientists use them.

In engineering, stress is a measure of how much pressure any material can withstand without undergoing some sort of physical change. Strain is a measure of how much physical change – such as stretching or flattening – actually happens in the material in response to stress. So while we are all subject to stress, the real measure of how damaging this is to our health is strain.

Too much stress results in extreme strain; everything and everyone has a breaking point. We instinctively understand that, when we describe someone for whom the strain has become unbearable as having had a breakdown.

We want to help you develop your resilience to stress by becoming better able to cope and less likely to 'break down' – in effect to find ways to reduce the amount of strain you suffer in response to stress.

There are no hard and fast rules about how much stress causes strain – in the same way that materials vary in their breaking points, people also vary in their reactions. The strain we suffer is a function not only of the intensity of the stress but also of our perception of and reaction to the threat, and we now have a far greater understanding of why this is the case.

Different reactions to stress

Part of the reason why some of us react to stress more strongly than others lies in the way the brain stores memories associated with strong negative emotions such as fear, anger and disgust in the unconscious mind. When we encounter a sudden threat, the fast breathing, upset digestion and other unpleasant associations that we experience are registered and stored in the amygdala, which is the brain centre for unconscious memory as well as being our 'fear centre'. At the same time, the hormones that our bodies produce in response to stress shut down our conscious long-term and short-term memories so they temporarily stop functioning. The result is that we act and record the event only in the instinctive rapid-response part of the brain. This system evolved to enable our ancestors to respond as rapidly as possible to sudden threats but it is now thought that it is these powerful unconscious memories that can cause us to over-react to stress. For example, if as a child you witnessed violent arguments between your parents, you are likely to over-react to situations which your instinctive brain perceives as similar in adulthood. So it is not surprising that children who had responsive, affectionate and predictable parenting are generally more robust and secure as adults. Later in this chapter we will describe how these memory responses can be treated effectively so that strain is minimised.

The effects of strain

We explained in Step 2 how the changes that take place in the autonomic nervous system in response to stress can disturb our inner balance and cause strain. These changes were first described by the endocrinologist Hans Selye in 1936 when he showed that rats exposed to unpleasant stimuli, such as extreme cold or electric shocks, go through a similar series of reactions.[2] Recent observations have found that the same reactions occur in humans in similar situations.[3]

Selye outlined three stages in the stress response:

- Stage One : The alarm, or 'fight or flight', response.
- Stage Two: Ongoing stress which results in the body being exposed to excessive levels of stress hormones.

- Stage Three: The body becomes progressively depleted and eventually reaches a stage of mental and physical exhaustion – severe strain – as a result of chronic stress. Important physiological and biochemical changes are involved in severe strain but one of the most important involves cortisol.[4]

Cortisol is a necessary part of our stress response as well as being a key hormone that helps release energy, maintains the correct water balance in our bodies and counters inflammation and allergies. However, ongoing high levels of cortisol can interfere with our sleep, dampen our inflammatory and immune response, interfere with the action of the main neurotransmitters such as serotonin and switch on the amygdala. Chronic strain accompanied by high levels of circulating cortisol can affect our ability to cope and think logically. Recent evidence from Southwestern Biomedical Center, University of Texas in the US, has shown that chronic strain as a result of prolonged psychosocial stress can cause some people to over-eat because it increases levels of ghrelin – known as the 'hunger hormone'.[5]

The good news is that all the most recent research shows that we are not stuck with the impact of chronic stress – our mental state can be improved dramatically. This is because the brain has a property known as plasticity whereby it can not only grow new neurons from its own stem cells but also constantly rewires itself so it can effectively be remoulded.[6]

how to cope

Now we are going to tell you how to minimise the strain that results from the stress of your cancer diagnosis and from the other stressors in your life.

Coping with the stress of cancer

Your first reaction to a cancer diagnosis is likely to be fear and anxiety. This is absolutely normal – cancer is probably the most-feared disease and it would be strange if people affected by cancer did not feel frightened and anxious.[7] Although your GP or oncologist might suggest medication, particularly if you suffer from insomnia, we would advise you to try to avoid taking tranquillisers such as benzodiazepines, if you can. The long-term use of these drugs can cause addiction, make normal sleep almost impossible and make people more anxious than ever.[8] There are lots of other ways to cope which do not involve taking drugs and which can be far more helpful in the long term.

Talk about it

A cancer diagnosis has a ripple effect. As well as the impact that it has on you, your family and other loved ones may be anxious and distressed as well. Turning to your partner, family and friends for support might feel like the most natural thing to do. At the same time it is easy to feel overwhelmed by visits and phone calls and people wanting frequent updates on your health and treatment. It may be helpful to think about setting some ground rules that are right for you and the family and friends who are supporting you. Everyone is different but here are some suggestions:

- Please do not ask me how I am every day.
- I will tell you if there are any changes.
- Please do not give me any advice unless I ask for it.
- Please do not tell me about someone else you know with the same condition especially if this is a scary story.

Sometimes it can be hard to confide in the people closest to you because you want to protect them from your worst fears. In this case it can help to talk to someone who is professionally trained to deal with the problems you face. Many hospitals now offer psychological support to cancer patients in the form of counselling, cognitive behavioural therapy (CBT) and/or psychodynamic therapy (PDT), so ask your nurse about the availability of such help. As well as hospitals' own services there are now 21 *Maggie's Centres* attached to hospitals around the UK. Named after their co-founder Maggie Keswick Jencks, a writer and artist who died of breast cancer in 1995, the centres provide free practical and emotional support for as long as it is needed for cancer patients, their family members and friends.

Many local cancer-support centres such as the Sutton Coldfield Cancer Support Centre and the Wirral Holistic Centre established by the wonderful Dorothy Crowther, a former NHS nurse, offer free or low-cost complementary therapies and counselling. Other centres provide support for particular cancer types such as The Haven which specialises in helping people with breast cancer. Jane and her friend Laura Jones run a website and hotline for cancer patients.[9] Mustafa also runs a drop-in centre for cancer patients in north London called The Amber Care Centre.

Coping with life stressors

As we have learnt, it is not the acute one-off incidents, such as a big row with your partner, that cause strain, it is the ongoing chronic stress. Whether you have a cancer diagnosis or not, it makes sense to try to deal with as many of these as possible. The knowledge that a partner has been unfaithful, the loss of a loved one through bereavement or divorce, unemployment or the ongoing pressures of being a carer can all cause serious strain.[10] The crisis of a cancer diagnosis can throw these issues into sharp focus and highlight the need to address them. For some people cancer can feel like a wake-up call – a chance to review their life, to mend difficult relationships with family or friends and to let go of past grievances.

Finding the support you need

In some cases practical support, such as effective respite for carers of seriously ill patients, can help, but for many people talking therapies are the best way to address these issues. Talking things through with a counsellor or therapist who can help you find your way forward can be enormously helpful.

The type of therapy you choose will depend on what feels right for you. If your problems are rooted in a difficult childhood you may find psychodynamic therapy most helpful. This aims to help us to understand and move on from the coping patterns we developed as children. Cognitive behavioural therapy, on the other hand, is a short-term therapy which focuses on 'reframing' our thoughts and behaviours to enable us to change the way we respond to problems.[11]

There used to be long waiting lists for these treatments, for patients who could not afford to pay, but facilities for cancer patients are becoming more widely available in both the NHS and the voluntary sector. So a diagnosis of cancer means that now is the time to deal with any old or long-term problems that are undermining your health.

Of course, not everyone wants to see a counsellor. If you are religious you might find it helpful to talk to a priest or a similar person of another faith. There are also many self-help books aimed at helping to resolve serious life problems. We list some examples in the Resources section at the end of this book.

Dealing with insomnia

Many cancer patients experience insomnia long after their cancer treatment is over – and stress plays a big role in this. The two graphs overleaf (Figure 8.1) represent heart-rate variability in the same person at rest, while experiencing different emotional states. The first shows what can happen when you get into bed tired and stressed – and then get even more tired and stressed about not being able to sleep. As you get more stressed and frustrated, your sympathetic nervous system is activated, reducing regular heart-rate variability.

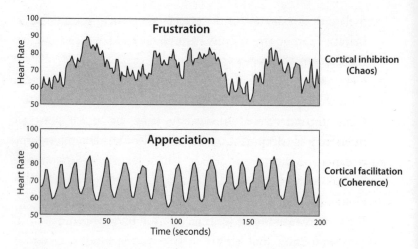

Figure 8.1 *Heart-rate variability. The bottom graph is far more balanced than the top, and it also shows a stronger variation between two beats.*

There is a close connection between serotonin, the so-called 'feel-good' neurotransmitter, and melatonin, the hormone produced by the pineal gland in response to darkness. Some serotonin is transformed into melatonin, and this creates physiological tiredness. Melatonin levels are increased by positive emotions and sufficient darkness, helping to induce and maintain sleep. Melatonin thereby helps to bring and maintain a state of rejuvenation and regeneration.

Once you start having problems sleeping it can rapidly become a vicious cycle. You go to bed feeling anxious, and then lie awake worrying about the fact that you are unable to sleep.

If you are worried about your sleep patterns talk to your doctor or nurse about it and try these self-help measures:

- Try to maintain a regular pattern of going to bed and getting up at the same time each day.
- Make sure that your bedroom is quiet, comfortably warm and dark. Light, whether it is daylight or artificial light, can suppress

melatonin production and hamper sleep. Some people find it helpful to wear the sort of eye covers that are given out for night flights by aircraft staff.

- Get some regular exercise during the day if you can (see Step 6). Even a short walk can help improve the quality of your sleep.
- Pain, discomfort and medication such as steroids can all interfere with sleep. If these are a problem talk to your doctor or cancer nurse.
- Try not to sleep for too long during the day as this can hinder night-time sleep.
- If you are awake for longer than 20 minutes get up and go into another room – do not go back to bed until you feel sleepy.
- Avoid stimulants such as tea or coffee which can affect sleep quality, close to bedtime. Also, some foods can affect sleeping habits, so keeping a personal food diary can help.
- If you tend to lie awake worrying, keep a notebook to write down your worries before you go to bed. You can come back to them in the morning and talk them through with someone who can help.
- Try diaphragm breathing and body scan meditation which can be very calming and particularly helpful in getting to sleep. Ensure that you are in a quiet, dark room and that your phone is switched off. Sit or lie down, ensuring that you are comfortable, and place your hands, one on top of the other, just below your navel. As you breathe you should notice your hands go up when you breathe in, and down as you breathe out. Breathing in this way will ensure that you are using your diaphragm which is calming. If you take lots of short, shallow breaths it signals anxiety to your brain.

Coping with practical problems

A cancer diagnosis and treatment plan will almost inevitably mean that you need some time off work, so it is important to make use of the help that is available. If you are not being given the time off that you need for treatment or recovery, or if you feel bullied or pressurised at work, talk your problems through with someone trained to deal with such situations. You need to find someone who is discreet and knowledgeable who can advise and support you. If your company has a human resources department they should be able to help. Alternatively contact your local Citizens' Advice Bureau (CAB) or Macmillan Cancer Support which provides employment information and advice to people with cancer.

Cancer can create serious financial problems for some people and debt can cause serious strain. If you are in financial difficulties because of cancer, or if debt is a major stressor in your life, try to address it as soon as possible. Your local CAB has trained advisors who can offer free, confidential, impartial and independent advice at more than 3,500 locations throughout the UK. They can be found on high streets, as well as in community centres, doctors' surgeries, courts and prisons.

The CAB not only helps people resolve debt issues, but also problems with benefits, employment, housing, discrimination and many more issues. However difficult your situation feels, seeking help and talking it through can only improve things and the sooner you do this the lower your strain will become.

Take control

One of the hardest things about a cancer diagnosis is feeling that you have lost control – so here is some advice about taking control. First you need to get the best conventional treatment you can find, with a medical team that you feel comfortable with and that you trust (see Step 3). If there are occasions when you feel you would like a second opinion, talk to your health team. A good oncologist, with the best interests of their patient at heart, will understand, respect and support this. In general, however, running around getting many different medical opinions is unhelpful, especially if this involves extra expense paying private doctors and therapists.

If you do want a second opinion, make sure the doctor works or has worked in the NHS.

Many cancer patients spend hours on the internet reading about their condition, some of which can be very frightening. Bear in mind that information (and misinformation) can be freely posted on the internet and some of it will be placed there by unscrupulous operators trying to sell you something. We generally recommend against this sort of activity – see also the box on page 86.

There are now dozens of books aimed at cancer patients, many of them about diet and of variable quality. Some contain information that is based on old wives' tales and half-understood science. The books we recommend are listed under the Resources section (see page 241).

Responding to stress

The role of stress (including both eustress – good stress – and distress) has been used to understand heart disease since 1974, based on the human function curve (Figure 8.2, overleaf). This is a way of illustrating the relationship between the person and the effects of the strain he or she experiences. It was first developed by Richard Lazarus, an American psychologist who was a pioneer in the study of stress.[12] It helps us to visualise our situation and our levels of stress and strain. The horizontal axis represents stress and the vertical axis strain. It is interesting to note that the curve shows that lack of stress is as harmful as too much, which explains why isolation and loneliness are so damaging. In fact, there is evidence that stress up to a point can be good.[13] This is the kind of stress that will be involved in achieving something worthwhile, meeting a realistic deadline and seeing the product and feeling good about the end result. All these can be uplifting and beneficial for health.

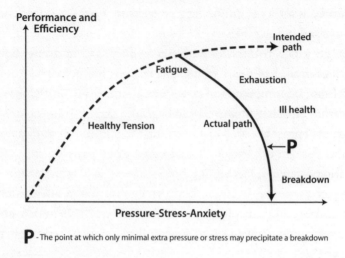

P - The point at which only minimal extra pressure or stress may precipitate a breakdown

Figure 8.2 *Human function curve.*

Look after yourself

Our bodies have a basic rest–activity cycle. When we need a rest, our bodies send us clear signals such as fidgetiness, hunger, drowsiness, and loss of focus. We usually condition ourselves to ignore and override these signals, resulting in a rise in our adrenalin and cortisol levels (which is particularly unhelpful at night when we need to sleep).

If we operate at high intensity for more than 90 minutes, we are likely to move from parasympathetic to sympathetic arousal – the physiological state more commonly known as 'fight or flight'. Taking breaks every 90 minutes, as much as you can, will automatically help your body get back to its natural rhythm of recovery.

Use mind-body techniques to reduce strain

These methods aim to work through our emotional brain (see Steps 2 and 4). Exercise (Step 6) is one of the most powerful ways to reduce strain, as is being part of a social network. For disabled or housebound people this can mean using the internet to join a social network, as a way of connecting with other people. Volunteering is an excellent way for those without family or close friends to establish a network that lowers strain. There are some excellent charities in the UK that offer the chance to connect people.[14]

Mind-body approaches to reducing strain can be extremely powerful, especially if you practise them regularly. They include a range of approaches such as music (singing, playing an instrument or just listening), yoga, acupuncture and acupressure, and emotional freedom technique whereby patients learn to tap on a sequence of acupuncture points while making an affirmation. Mindfulness and meditation are also extremely helpful[15] and brain-scanning studies have shown that they are effective in calming the mind and reducing strain.[16] Jane attends a weekly Sangha meeting where mindful meditation is practised. Gaia House and the Community of Interbeing UK organise Sangha around the country (see Resources). It is a matter of looking at what is on offer and finding the approach that works for you – it does not have to be complicated. Simply spending time in a green (or blue) space can be restorative. A walk in a park, a trip to the country or seaside, exploring beautiful gardens – all are natural, cheap and, research has confirmed, very effective.[17]

Helpful books, websites and organisations are listed in the Resources section at the end of this book.

step 9
broaden your awareness

Now you are nearing the end of this book and know more about how to protect yourself against cancer, you may be wondering why no one has given you this breadth and depth of information about cancer before. Here, we aim to broaden your awareness by explaining to you why doctors, charities and the media may be constrained in the information they provide. We believe that this will empower you further to make the best decisions in preventing and treating cancer.

Your immediate question will be why is the information to be given here – which we regard as essential for everyone facing cancer – not made more widely available? The answer is that the priorities of modern healthcare and its providers are complicated, especially in the cancer field. Money and politics permeate every aspect of the system – and cancer, like the rest of healthcare, is no exception. Think back to the battles over Herceptin. It was hailed as a breakthrough drug and the first effective treatment for women with HER2 positive breast cancer – but some local NHS bodies refused to pay for it. A huge public row ensued in which the then Health Secretary intervened on behalf of patients. The same scenario has been enacted multiple times since then.

Cancer is big business. Drugs mean big profits for manufacturers, distributors, lobbyists and PR agencies! When the stakes are so high it is hardly surprising that the voices of those who advocate prevention as well as cure are difficult to hear. Of course, it takes years and billions of pounds' worth of investment to develop, test and market a new drug.[1] In the process, many candidates fail. It can be said, with only slight exaggeration, that to treat the first patient with a new product costs billions, whereas treatment for the second patient may only cost a few pounds. How the cost of treating this first patient should be spread among subsequent patients is a legitimate subject for debate. Companies naturally want to recover their investment and make as much profit as soon as possible, but the price of a drug does not always reflect its production cost, and its availability may vary from one area to another.

While organisations like cancer-research charities, medical research institutions and healthcare providers are not commercial in the same way as pharmaceutical companies, they are subject to similar pressures. Some are wealthy, others less so, but most have massive budgets. They all have to raise finance from public and philanthropic donations, government and private contracts, corporate and individual clients. Like commercial companies, cancer charities now employ sophisticated marketing techniques to raise money for their 'cause'. In the process, the real cancer message is invariably reduced to a soundbite, rather than telling people about the environmental and social changes needed to eliminate the root causes of the disease. Nowhere is this more clearly demonstrated than in the case of breast cancer and its pink ribbon campaign, begun in the USA by Estee Lauder Cosmetics.[2] Breast Cancer Awareness month with its trademark pink ribbons has become a powerful marketing tool not just for the cancer charities, but for everyone from bra manufacturers to leading supermarkets. While Estee Lauder has donated over $25 million to breast-cancer research, some companies have been exposed for misusing the pink ribbon – which is not actually licensed by any corporation – and donating little if any of their revenue to breast-cancer research. We recommend that before you donate to charities, you check out how much of their budget is devoted to actual research and/or practical support for cancer patients.

Charities, research institutions and healthcare providers also have to work with whoever is the government of the day. So they have to be seen to 'fit' the established way of thinking, talk the right language, and be wary of rocking any boats. Otherwise, they may see their funding dry up.

To some extent government and state institutions do well. Together with international agencies, the UK government has now banned or restricted many dangerous chemicals as evidence began to accumulate about their possible carcinogenic and other damaging effects. There are many more chemicals that have yet to be added to the banned and restricted list, and work is ongoing. The problem is that, inevitably, there is a time lag between the science and the decision to ban or restrict hazardous substances. Politicians and public officials may not have any expert understanding of science, medicine or the nature of evidence, so they do not always appreciate the significance of advice. What is more, their focus is often on the economics of business, rather than public interest and safety. That is particularly evident in connection with manufactured foods and the dairy industry which represent around 12 per cent of the UK's GDP. It is hardly surprising, therefore, that risks are sometimes ignored, at least until the consequences become obvious to everyone. Be in no doubt that here again vested interests in the form of powerful lobby groups are hard at work persuading the authorities that their products are safe and essential to modern life. So do not assume that whatever you buy must be safe. Follow the advice given in Step 7 on how to limit your exposure to carcinogens in the environment, and consult experts.

Ideas that may seem innovative are welcome up to a point, but not if they put important vested interests at risk or limit funds that may be better spent to get real effects and make a difference. Imagine a situation where a major shareholder or donor – nowadays often called a 'corporate partner' or a 'venture capitalist'

– is a company whose products contain chemicals recently found to be carcinogenic. Is it likely that funding would be provided for research that could demonstrate that these products were the cause of cancer in a significant percentage of real patients? And if the money were available, would the company be willing to do the research that would prove its own products contained carcinogenic chemicals?

Where there is money, there is also power and influence. Rich and powerful organisations can have direct access to politicians and government officials. They can afford to pay lobbyists who seek to influence national and EU legislation, and employ top PR companies who work wonders in persuading the media and others to accept their clients' views. The reality is that most people probably get most of their information from newspapers, television, radio, magazines and the internet. You probably know that the media are not necessarily always as objective as they would like us to believe. When the subject depends on specialist knowledge and expertise, it can become even more difficult for the general public to judge. Media coverage of cancer and related issues is like the traditional curate's egg: it is good in parts. There are some excellent and well-qualified science journalists whose writing illuminates difficult and tricky subjects. A key problem is that many reporters fail to ask scientists the crucial questions: 'Who is funding you and how does this research promote their interests?' Trained scientists would be able to distinguish between good and bad science and recognise vested interests at play. In contrast, it can be harder for editors, particularly those involved in light entertainment rather than serious scientific journalism, and for the general public.

Cancer is now such big business! Some commentators have described it as an 'industry': one that is vast and ever-expanding, more concerned with the orthodox management of the disease than prevention, preoccupied with new therapies and with research and financial investment for a burgeoning future market.[3] This trend is likely to continue since the latest (2014) statistics from the World Heath Organization (WHO) predict that 'Cancer cases worldwide are forecast to rise by 75 per cent and reach close to 25 million over the next two decades').[4]

We think that the commercial analysis goes too far, not least because advances in orthodox cancer treatment mean that many people are alive and flourishing today who, even 10 years ago, would have died. Nevertheless we agree with Dr Samuel Epstein, Professor of Environmental and Occupational Health at the University of Illinois, who has repeatedly highlighted the failings of the cancer establishment. In *Criminal Indifference to Cancer Prevention and Conflicts of Interest* he indicts the USA's National Cancer Institute and the American Cancer Society 'for their reckless indifference to cancer prevention, for their incestuous relationship with the cancer drug industry, and for their false claims for miracle cancer drugs and winning the war against cancer'.[5] Dr Epstein is similarly forthright about the role of vested interests in the chemical and associated industries that put the profit motive ahead of concern for human health.

He is certainly not alone. As you will have discovered in this book, many distinguished doctors and scientists have shown in their peer-reviewed writing and presentations how vested interests in the food industry manipulate politicians and others in the establishment. This confuses the public about the real causes of cancer. Evidence is clear that it is the Western diet, full of animal-based foods such as meat and dairy and refined and processed food, that is a large part of the problem.

Today, there is general agreement on some issues concerning the prevention and treatment of cancer, especially the benefits of exercise and the hazards and risks of smoking. Some progress is being made on recognising the importance of diet. Organisations such as the World Cancer Research Fund and WHO, for example, are increasingly emphasising that a good diet can cut cancer risk by 30–40 per cent. While there is still controversy about 'anti-cancer' diets and about limiting exposure to harmful substances in the environment, the new science of 'epigenetics' is proving beyond any doubt that these can work, right down to our genes (Steps 1, 5 and 7). Nevertheless, if you go generally 'looking', you are unlikely to get anything but the most general advice from the majority of cancer charities or health professionals. We believe that if you rely solely on the cancer prevention advice from government, charities, health professionals or the media you will be missing out on vital and potentially life-saving information. In this book, we have aimed to empower you with the right choices and the direction to take.

Most of us take it for granted that health professionals are experts on everything to do with health. That is simply unrealistic. While many – particularly those cancer specialists who are research-active – provide excellent advice on the orthodox management of cancer, few are experts in nutrition. The biochemistry of how our bodies process the food we eat is complex, yet medical training contains little, if any, nutritional biochemistry. With such limited knowledge of expert science, perhaps it is not surprising that many doctors and dietitians continue to reject the role of diet as part of cancer treatment. Worse, they may even recommend foods that have been shown to promote cancer by leading researchers in the best universities in the world.

Where does all of this leave those of you, like Jane, who live with cancer in their daily lives? We hope that it will be the catalyst that makes you determined to inform yourself as widely as possible – and develop a healthy scepticism about advice that comes from vested interests. Whenever money is involved, someone may have a motive to adapt their advice to protect their income.

We believe strongly that when it comes to the prevention of cancer our life is still, to a great extent, in our own hands. We must decide for ourselves what information we need, whether to trust it – and who is out for personal gain or glory and who is telling the truth. We have to be ready to consider changing our lifestyles to minimise the risk of cancer. Realistically, it is impossible to eliminate cancer risks completely in the modern world, but that should not stop us from giving ourselves the best possible chance.

Your doctors and medical team are well placed to give you the best advice about treatments and care, and send you in the right direction. However, they are unlikely to be expert in either nutritional biochemistry or the risks posed by hazardous substances in the environment. For sound information on these, you will need to go to experts elsewhere and we hope that this book and the references it contains will give you a good start.

We firmly believe in an integrated approach to cancer treatment. Dedicated biomedical scientists continue to make major advances in increasing the efficacy of treatments while reducing their side effects. Conventional medicine can be made much more effective by integrating it with other scientifically based approaches. Based upon evidence, we believe that these include adopting the anti-cancer diet proposed here and by developing personal exercise regimens and stress-management techniques. Jane has kept her cancer genes under control now for more than 25 years – over one-third of her life – and has helped others to do the same. She has refused to be a cancer victim. She has simply worked with her health professionals who are among the best in the world while she takes charge of everything else to do with her health. In this book we have given you the information that will enable you to do the same. We have provided you with all the very latest evidence-based scientific information on cancer, including hot-off-the-press information from Mustafa's world-leading laboratories, to help you to take your life firmly into your own hands.

step 10
stay on course

This chapter is short but nevertheless it is very important. You have survived cancer. You might have had surgery, almost certainly chemotherapy, maybe radiotherapy and possibly other treatments too. You may have gone through one of the most difficult and distressing periods of your life. Now it is time to move on to the next stage. Hopefully, your cancer is in remission. For some of you, this means the end of treatment, while others – particularly those whose cancer was hormone related – will continue with drug therapies to stop the cancer returning. Alternatively, your cancer might be under control but there is a possibility you might need further treatment in the future. Whichever group you fall into, congratulations! You deserve to celebrate the good news, but it is also important that you remain vigilant!

Most people at this point want to know how to stay healthy. If you feel vulnerable or worried about the cancer recurring and cannot imagine how to get back to normal life, be reassured firstly that this is perfectly natural. While few people are sorry to complete their treatment, it is not unusual to miss the hospital routine or the reassurance of ongoing medical care. You may feel strangely bereft at the loss of your regular appointments with health professionals. The thought of taking back responsibility for your own health can be daunting and feel frightening. Left to yourself you may notice every ache and pain, feel panicked when you see something about cancer and find that your confidence is at a low ebb. Almost all cancer survivors feel like this once the euphoria has passed but it is part of the process of recovery. Be reassured that, in time, you will move on from these feelings.

Nobody can guarantee that your cancer will not return, but there is a great deal that you can do to reduce your risk. Just as importantly, taking these steps will help to keep you fit and healthy – and so best equipped to fight off other illnesses as well.

There are two things that are important to understand. First, having being touched by cancer means that your body has some kind of susceptibility, which is likely to remain for the rest of your life. So getting back to normal life means discovering what is your new 'normal'. It may or may not be the same as it was before your cancer. Second, the external environment and its inherent health risks are unlikely to improve much in the foreseeable future. So as well as managing your diet (Step 5) and working to stay healthy follow our suggestions in Steps 6, 7 and 8.

It is not until you experience cancer that you realise that life is always a balance between pro-cancer and anti-cancer effects. Armed with the information in this book, you can now take steps to ensure that the anti-cancer effects outweigh the pro-cancer ones as much as possible and for as long as possible (Figure 10.1, below).

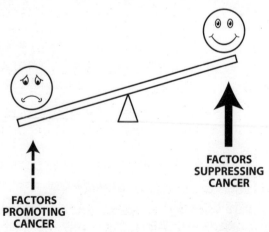

Figure 10.1 *Living with cancer is possible if the factors suppressing cancer outweigh those factors that promote it.*

protect yourself

Keep taking your medication

Many cancer patients are given long-term drug treatment – often to help prevent the cancer recurring. For example, people with hormonal cancers, such as breast or prostate cancer, may be given drug treatment to prevent hormones promoting their cancer. Some people experience unpleasant side effects from the drugs. If this is the case for you, talk to your oncologist who may be able to change the dose or type of drug since often there are alternatives. Never just stop taking your medication without discussing it with your oncologist.

Be alert to any changes

You know your body best and can monitor it from day to day and notice anything that does not seem right. Cancers do sometimes come back. For example, one in five of breast cancer cases will return after treatment within a few years. So, it is important to be alert to any worrying changes. With any cancer, take unexplained symptoms (listed in Step 3) that last more than a few weeks seriously. Having said that, it is important to find a balance between being alert to changes and constantly worrying about the cancer coming back. If the cancer does come back, please do not feel it is the end of the world, or that it is, somehow, your fault. It is likely that some undetectable microscopic disease may have remained after your treatment and can be treated again. Many people have survived cancer more than once and it is possible to live with cancer.

Keep in touch with your oncologist

If you do have worrying symptoms, your first port of call will probably be your GP. Family doctors vary enormously in their approach, especially with the limited time (currently, 10 minutes) they have for appointments. Whatever your GP's response, if you are still worried, insist that thorough tests are carried out. It is always better to be safe than sorry. During your treatment, try and establish a rapport with your oncologist and remain in touch, even from a distance. If you are worried that your cancer may be back, ask to see an oncologist as soon as possible, ideally the same oncologist who treated you (Figure 10.2, below).

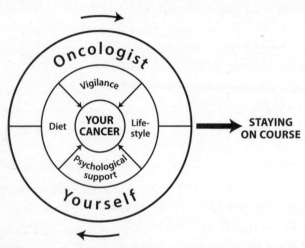

Figure 10.2 *You and your oncologist together, through vigilance, diet and lifestyle with psychological support, will enable you to keep the cancer under control and stay on course, both during and following your treatment.*

Eat a healthy diet

As we demonstrated in Step 5, we really are what we eat. Our diet has a major impact on our body chemistry which, in turn, affects everything from major bodily functions like digestion to more subtle aspects such as our mood. Alongside all this is the potential involvement of 'epigenetics'. Although research in this area is in its infancy there is increasing evidence that diet can directly affect the expression levels of our genes, including cancer genes. For example, eating raw spinach has been shown to suppress those genes driving the invasiveness in colon cancer.[1]

Maintain a healthy weight

It is almost impossible to open a newspaper or watch TV news these days without hearing about the obesity epidemic. Obesity is a risk factor for many types of cancer. However, some cancer patients have the opposite problem – having lost a lot of weight when they were ill, they now need to gain it. We explained the essentials of what you need to do to maintain a healthy weight in Step 5 but you may also need the help and support of a qualified dietitian. Nevertheless, always question the advice you are given and remain critical. Also remember that being skinny does not necessarily mean you are unhealthy. There is strong evidence that calorie restriction prolongs life. Note that many vegans can appear skinny – for example the recently converted Bill Clinton.

Keep active

As we saw in Step 6, being active is important both in protecting against cancer and in helping your recovery. The good news is that it is never too late to start. Even people who start exercising late in life gain many of the same health benefits as those who have exercised all their lives. It can be hard to get going, especially if you feel tired and low after treatment, but once you get moving you will find that exercise has significant psychological as well as physical benefits. It can lift your mood, boost your energy levels and really help in your journey back to 'normal life'. You can start small, with a short walk every day, and gradually build up or if that is not possible do some simple stretching and toning exercises at home. If your physiotherapist has given you exercises to help build up muscle mass, do them religiously. It will not be long before you feel the benefits.

getting back to work

If you have surgery you will certainly have to take time off work and although some people continue working during chemotherapy or radiotherapy, many need to take sick leave. At some point, you will start thinking about getting back to work. Going back to work after cancer treatment can feel daunting for all sorts of reasons – while financial pressures might mean you need to return as early as possible.

Although most employers are supportive, there are always some who are less co-operative. The good news is that under the 2010 Equality Act,* anyone with a cancer diagnosis has a right to what are called 'reasonable adjustments'. These might include time off for medical appointments, a gradual, phased return to work, being flexible about working hours or offering the opportunity to work from home some of the time. The new Act also protects you against discrimination, victimisation or harassment. For instance, employers can no longer ask questions about your health at job interviews (although it is lawful to do so for monitoring purposes). Importantly, the new Act now protects carers against discrimination, although it does not require the employer to offer 'reasonable adjustments'.

If you feel you are not being treated fairly at work, talk to the human resources department if there is one, your trade union, the Citizens' Advice Bureau or one of the patient-support organisations (see Resources page 242). All these organisations should be able to advise and offer practical support. Macmillan Cancer Support has a useful, free tool to help you sort out what questions you need to ask about returning to work and where to get the answers.[2] Concerns about money can also be a major headache for cancer patients and their families. If you are employed you should be covered by your organisation's sick-pay scheme.

---

* This replaced the old Disability Discrimination Act (DDA) in England, Scotland and Wales. If you live in Northern Ireland, the DDA still applies.

ask for help when you need it

Having cancer is a life-changing experience! This is the time when you may feel in most need of support. The first stop could be your doctor. He or she may be able to help with both physical and psychological symptoms. But medical support is often not enough. Although your family and friends will be supportive, it can sometimes be difficult for those closest to you to know how to help. Everyone is different but finding the support of a counsellor, a cancer 'buddy' or a support group can all help (see Resources). If you feel anxious find ways to relax and deal with stress and strain – mindfulness training, meditation and other complementary therapies can be particularly helpful. There are many groups and patient organisations that offer genuinely helpful support. Your doctor may know of such local groups, or you could search online. You may also need to access welfare benefits and, if you need advice, your trade union or local Citizens' Advice Bureau should be able to help. Macmillan Cancer Support's helpline will be able to put you in touch with one of their welfare rights advisers.

live your life!

Now that you have completed your treatment, you have the chance to take stock of your life and decide how to move forward in the best way. For many people the experience of cancer leads to very positive changes. As hard as it is to go through cancer, many survivors say it has enabled them to grow – to appreciate life, to value their families and friends more, even to take up new interests or perhaps find a new career. Wherever you are on this journey, you have our very best wishes. Enjoy your life.

appendix

Table A: Alkali-generating and acid-generating foods*

	-20 Very strongly alkaline	-10 Strongly alkaline	-5 Alkaline	-0.5 Moderately alkaline
Herbs and spices	Parsley, dried -62.4	Curry powder -19.9	-	Chives -3.6
	Basil, dried -57.9	Black pepper -19.7	-	-
	Ginger -23	-	-	-
Fruits and juices	Raisins -21	-	Blackcurrants -6.5	Apricots -4.8
	-	-	Bananas -5.5	Kiwi fruit -4.1
	-	-	-	Tomato juice -3.8
	-	-	-	Cherries -3.6
	-	-	-	Orange juice -2.9
	-	-	-	Pears -2.9
	-	-	-	Oranges -2.7
	-	-	-	Pineapple -2.7
	-	-	-	Lemon juice -2.5
	-	-	-	Peaches -2.4
	-	-	-	Apple juice -2.2

* The chart included here is based on the work of two distinguished biochemists at the Institute of Clinical Nutrition in Dortmund, Germany who used computer models and experimental animal and finally human studies to determine the Renal Acid Load left to be excreted by the kidney after food is metabolised.

0 Nearly neutral	0.5 Moderately acid	5 Acid	10 Strongly acid	20 Very strongly acid
-	-	-	-	-
-	-	-	-	-
-	-	-	-	-
	-	-	-	-
-	-	-	-	-
-	-	-	-	-
-	-	-	-	-
-		-	-	-
-	-	-	-	-
-	-	-	-	-
-	-	-	-	-
-	-	-	-	-
-	-	-	-	-
-	-	-	-	-

	-20 Very strongly alkaline	-10 Strongly alkaline	-5 Alkaline	-0.5 Moderately alkaline
Fruit and juices (cont'd)	-	-	-	Apples -2.2
	-	-	-	Strawberries -2.2
	-	-	-	Watermelon -1.9
Vegetables	-	Spinach -14	Celery -5.2	Carrots, young -4.9
	-	-	-	Courgette -4.6
	-	-	-	Cauliflower -4.0
	-	-	-	Potatoes, old -4.0
	-	-	-	Radish, red -3.7
	-	-	-	Aubergine -3.4
	-	-	-	Tomatoes -3.1
	-	-	-	Beans, green -3.1
	-	-	-	Lettuce -2.5
	-	-	-	Chicory -2.0
	-	-	-	Leeks -1.8
	-	-	-	Lettuce, iceberg -1.6
	-	-	-	Onions -1.5
	-	-	-	Mushrooms -1.4

0 Nearly neutral	0.5 Moderately acid	5 Acid	10 Strongly acid	20 Very strongly acid
-	-	-	-	-
-	-	-	-	-
-	-	-	-	-
Asparagus -0.4	-	-	-	-
-	-	-	-	-
-	-	-	-	-
-	-	-	-	-
-	-	-	-	-
-	-	-	-	-
-	-	-	-	-
-	-	-	-	-
-	-	-	-	-
-	-	-	-	-
-	-	-	-	-
-	-	-	-	-
-	-	-	-	-

	-20 Very strongly alkaline	-10 Strongly alkaline	-5 Alkaline	-0.5 Moderately alkaline
	-	-	-	Peppers -1.4
	-	-	-	Broccoli -1.2
	-	-	-	Cucumber -0.8
Beverages	-	-	-	Red wine -2.4
	-	-	-	Mineral water -1.8
	-	-	-	Coffee -1.4
	-	-	-	White wine, dry -1.2
	-	-	-	Grape juice -1
	-	-	-	-
Fats and oils	-	-	-	-
	-	-	-	-
	-	-	-	-
Sugars, sweets and preserves	-	-	-	Marmalade -1.5
	-	-	-	-
Legumes and nuts	-	-	Soya flour -5.9	Soya beans -4.7

0 Nearly neutral	0.5 Moderately acid	5 Acid	10 Strongly acid	20 Very strongly acid
-	-	-	-	-
-	-	-	-	-
-	-	-	-	-
Cocoa -0.4	Beer, pale 0.9	-	-	-
Tea -0.3	-	-	-	-
Beer, draught -0.2	-	-	-	-
Beer, stout -0.1	-	-	-	-
Mineral water -0.1	-	-	-	-
Cola -0.4	-	-	-	-
Margarine -0.5	-	-	-	-
Olive oil 0.0	-	-	-	-
Sunflower-seed oil 0.0	-	-	-	-
Honey -0.3	Chocolate milk 2.4	-	-	-
Sugar, white -0.1	Madeira cake 3.7	-	-	-
Soya milk -0.3	Peas 1.2	Miso 6.9	-	-

	-20 Very strongly alkaline	-10 Strongly alkaline	-5 Alkaline	-0.5 Moderately alkaline
	-	-	-	Natto -3.2
	-	-	-	Hazelnuts -2.8
	-	-	-	-
	-	-	-	-
Grain products	-	-	-	-
	-	-	-	-
	-	-	-	-
	-	-	-	-
	-	-	-	-
	-	-	-	-
	-	-	-	-
	-	-	-	-
Meat	-	-	-	-
	-	-	-	-
	-	-	-	-

0 Nearly neutral	0.5 Moderately acid	5 Acid	10 Strongly acid	20 Very strongly acid
Soya bean, sprouted, raw 0.3	Mori-Nu tofu 2.0	Tempeh 8.2	-	-
	Tofu 3.4	Tofu, prepared with calcium sulphate 8.3	-	-
	Lentils 3.5	Walnuts 6.8	-	-
	Soya sauce 4.5	Peanuts, plain 8.3	-	-
	Rice, white, boiled 1.7	Rye flour, whole 5.9	Oat flakes 10.7	-
	Bread, wheat wholemeal 1.8	Cornflakes 6.0	Rice, brown 12.5	-
	Crisp bread, rye 3.3	Noodles, egg 6.4	-	-
	Bread, wheat, white 3.7	Spaghetti, white 6.5	-	-
	Bread, wheat, mixed 3.8	Wheat flour, white 6.9	-	-
	Bread, rye, mixed 4.0	Spaghetti, wholemeal 7.3	-	-
	Bread, rye 4.1	Wheat flour, wholemeal 8.2	-	-
	Rice, white 4.6	-	-	-
	-	Frankfurters 6.7	Luncheon meat 10.2	-
	-	Beef, lean 7.8	Liver sausage 10.6	-
	-	Pork, lean 7.9	Salami 11.6	-

	-20 Very strongly alkaline	-10 Strongly alkaline	-5 Alkaline	-0.5 Moderately alkaline
	-	-	-	-
	-	-	-	-
	-	-	-	-
	-	-	-	-
Fish and eggs	-	-	-	-
	-	-	-	-
	-	-	-	-
	-	-	-	-
Dairy products	-	-	-	-
	-	-	-	-
	-	-	-	-
	-	-	-	-
	-	-	-	-
	-	-	-	-
	-	-	-	-

0 Nearly neutral	0.5 Moderately acid	5 Acid	10 Strongly acid	20 Very strongly acid
-	-	Chicken, meat 8.7	Corned beef 13.2	-
-	-	Steak, lean and fat 8.8	-	-
-	-	Veal 9.0	-	-
-	-	Turkey, meat 9.9	-	-
-	Egg whites 1.1	Haddock 6.8	Trout 10.8	Egg yolks 23.4
-	-	Herring 7.0	-	-
-	-	Cod 7.1	-	-
-	-	Eggs, whole 8.2	-	-
-	Butter 0.6	Cottage cheese 8.7	Fresh cheese 11.1	Cheese, Cheddar-type, reduced fat 26.4
-	Ice cream 0.6	-	Camembert 14.6	Processed cheese 28.7
-	Milk, whole 0.7	-	Cheese, Gouda 18.6	Parmesan 34.2
-	Milk, evaporated 1.1	-	Hard cheese 19.2	-
-	Creams, fresh, sour 1.2	-	-	-
-	Yoghurt, fruit 1.2	-	-	-
-	Yoghurt, plain 1.5	-	-	-
	Soft cheese 4.3			

Table B: Concentrations of steroid oestrogens in various environmental matrices and foods

Environment	Oestrone (E1)	Oestradiol (E2)	Oestriol (E3)
Land sources (µg/kg)			
Soil	0.012–0.025	0.002–0.055	nd–0.001
Sewage sludge	5.6–25.2	1.7–5.1	
Swine manure	217–4,728	nd–1,215	
Dairy wastes	203–543	113–236	
Poultry manure	nd	14–904	
Aquatic environment (µg/L)			
Headwater stream	0.0001–0.009	nd–0.0009	nd
Surface water	nd–0.112	nd–0.200	nd–0.051
Groundwater	nd–0.120	nd–0.045	
Sea	nd–0.002		
Rain	nd	nd	
Food (µg/kg)			
Fish muscle	<0.02	<0.03	
Beef	nd–3.96	nd–1.03	
Dairy	0.01–1.47	0.01–0.09	
Pork	<26.06	nd–10.56	
Poultry	<0.02–0.51	nd–0.73	
Eggs	0.18–0.89	nd–0.22	
Vegetables	<0.01–0.02	nd	
Drinking water (g/L)	0.0002–0.0006	nd–0.002	nd

Table C: Food sources of phytochemicals and proposed mechanisms of action

Phytochemical	Food	Proposed mechanism(s) of action
Alkaloids		
Pyrrolidine dithiocarbamate	Leaves of tobacco and carrots	Inhibits NFkappaB to prevent cancer cachexia
Capsaicinoids		
Capsaicin	Chilli peppers	Modulation of cell signalling pathways through inhibition of phase I enzymes
[6-Gingerol]	Ginger	Inhibits VEGF and bFGF induced proliferation of human endothelial cells. Causes cell cycle arrest in G1 phase
Diterpenes		
Taxol	Yew tree	Used to treat ovarian, breast and non-small cell lung cancer
Phenanthroindolizidine alkaloid		
Tylophorine	Tylophoraindica plants	Down regulates cyclin A2, which plays an important role in G1 arrest in carcinoma cells
Purine alkaloids		
Methylxanthines (theophylline, theobromine, caffeine)	Coffee and tea	cAMP-phosphodiesterase inhibitors, involving alterations in cAMP system tumour cell
Vinca alkaloids		
Vinblastine, vincristine and vindesine	Vinca rosea	Potent microtubule destabilising agents first recognised for their myelosuppressive effects

Phytochemical	Food	Proposed mechanism(s) of action
Pentacyclic alkaloid		
Camptothecin	Camptotheca acuminata Decne	Antitumour activity from inhibiting the nuclear enzyme DNA topoisomerase
Carotenoids		
Fucoxanthin, peridinin	Brown seaweed	Anticarcinogenic properties
Lutein and Zeaxanthin	Dark green leafy vegetables, egg yolk	Selective modulation of apoptosis and inhibition of angiogenesis
Lycopene	Tomatoes, watermelon	Antioxidant
Neoxanthin, fucoxanthin	Spinach and brown seaweed	Reduces the proliferation of prostate-cancer cells
Phytofluene, carotene, lycopene	Tomatoes	Reduces the proliferation of prostate-cancer cells
Flavonoids		
Beta-carotene	Mangos, papayas, carrots, yams, spinach and kales	Inhibition of cyclooxygenase-2 enzymatic activity
Flavones		
Apigenin and luteolin	Artichokes	Stimulates enzymes that detoxify carcinogens
Luteolin	Apple skin, celery	Induction of apoptosis, and inhibition of cell proliferation, metastasis and angiogenesis

Phytochemical	Food	Proposed mechanism(s) of action
Flavanols		
Fisetin	Onion, cucumber, apple and strawberry	Inhibition of cyclooxygenase-2 enzymatic activity
Quercetin	Ginkgo leaves	Antioxidant, antilipoperoxidative properties, apoptosis of cancer cells
	Fruit, vegetables, tea and wine	Down regulating the expression of oncogenes (H-ras, c-myc and K-ras) and anti-oncogenes
	Onions	Modulation of cell signalling pathways, inhibition of COX-2, 5-LOX, 12-LOX and PLA2 enzymes
	Grape extracts (Cabernet Franc)	Induced mammalian phase II detoxification enzyme quinone reductase in Hepa1c1c7 murine hepatoma cells
Flavonols-catechins		
Epigallocatechin gallate (EGCG)	Green tea	Modulation of cell signalling pathways, anti-angiogenic, induction of apoptosis
Flavanones		
Hesperidin	Citrus fruits	Inhibits the proliferation of breast-cancer cells
Naringenin and bergamotin	Grapefruit juice	Inhibitors of phase I enzyme CYP3A4 in xenobiotic metabolism

Phytochemical	Food	Proposed mechanism(s) of action
Isoflavones		
Biochanin and genistein	Bean family	Inhibit the cell growth of stomach-cancer cells lines in vitro through activation of a signal transduction pathway for apoptosis
		Antioxidative and oestrogenic activity that has been reported to reduce the risk of breast cancer
Genistein	Grape extracts (Cabernet Franc)	Induced mammalian phase II detoxification enzyme quinone reductase in Hepa1c1c7 murine hepatoma cells
Organosulphur compounds		
Allicin	Garlic	Inhibits enzymes that activate cancer-causing chemicals inducing cell apoptosis
Diallyl sulphide & diallyl disulphide	Garlic	Cell arrest and apoptosis of cancer cells
Glucosinolate	Broccoli, cauliflower, Brussels sprouts	Potent inducers of phase II enzymes that protect against chemical carcinogens
Indole-3-carbinol	Cruciferous vegetables	Increase formation of antiproliferative oestradiol metabolite and induce cellular apoptosis
Isothiocyanates	Broccoli	Induction of phase II enzymes, modulation of cell signalling pathways, induction of apoptosis
Isothiocyanates	Broccoli, cauliflower, Brussels sprouts	Potent inducers of phase II enzymes that protect against chemical carcinogens
Phenylethylisothio-cyanate	Cruciferous vegetables	Induce apoptosis in human colon-cancer cell line HT-29 by activating the mitochondrial caspase cascade

Appendix

Phytochemical	Food	Proposed mechanism(s) of action
S-allyl-L-cysteine	Garlic	Antioxidant and inhibits enzymes that promote growth of tumours
Sulphoraphane	Cruciferous vegetables	Inhibition of adenoma formation in gastro-intestinal tract of mice from upregulation of pro-apoptotic genes including MBD4, TNF-7 and TNF(ligand)-11
Sulphoraphane	Cruciferous vegetables	Potent inducers of phase II enzymes that protect against chemical carcinogens

Phenolics

| *Anthraquinones* | Rhubarb, aloe, senna, purslane | Protective effects for the gastrointestinal and renal systems |

Hydroxy-benzoic acids

| Vanillin and gallic acid | Most plant leaves including those made into teas | Inhibition of Cyp2A2, 3A1, 2B2 and 2C6 in vitro |

Hydroxy-cinnamic acids

| Caffeic acid phenethly ester (CAPE) and ferulic acid | Coffee, honey | Induction of phase II enzymes |

Phenolic diarylheptanoids

| Yakuchinones A and B | Ginger (Alpinia oxyphylla) | Inhibits PMA-induced inflammation and epidermal ODC activity as well as skin-tumour promotion in female ICR mice |

Phytochemical	Food	Proposed mechanism(s) of action
Phytoalexin		
Resveratrol	Red grapes, red wine and peanuts	Modulation of cell signalling pathways, inhibition of angiogenesis and induction of apoptosis. Inhibits and retards tumour growth and cell growth arrest
Resveratrol	Grape extracts (Cabernet Franc)	Induced mammalian phase II detoxification enzyme quinone reductase in Hepa1c1c7 murine hepatoma cells
Polyphenols		
Anethole	Fennel and anise	Suppress NF-KB activation through the inhibition of IKB degradation
Curcumin	Turmeric	Inhibits tumour initiation by BaP and DMBA (dimethylbenz(a) anthracene) and also inhibits tumour promotion induced by 12-O-tetradecanoylphorbol-13-acetate (TPA)
Ellagic acid, ellagitannin, punicalagin	Pomegranate	Antiproliferative activity against oral, colon and prostate-cancer cells
Proanthocyanidin	Cocoa, grape skin, cranberry	Inhibition of matrix metalloproteinases, MMP-2 and MMP-9
Phyto-oestrogens		
Lignans	Flaxseed and grains	Prevents oestrogen and prostaglandin hormones from binding to their receptors (retarding cell proliferation)
Secoisolariciresinol diglucoside	Flax, sunflower, sesame and pumpkin seeds	Scavenging free radicals and inducing antioxidant enzymes (glutathione peroxidase and superoxide dismutase)

Phytochemical	Food	Proposed mechanism(s) of action
Spices		
Cinnamon extract	Food flavourings	Enhanced pro-apoptotic activity and inhibition of NFkappaB and AP1 activities and their target genes
Terpenoids		
Monoterpenes		
D-limonene	Orange peel and lemon peel	Inhibits neoplasia, stimulates enzymes that detoxify carcinogens, prevents expression of oncogenes
Triterpenoids		
Ginsenosides	Ginseng	Induce CYP3A4 and CYP2C9 enzymes anti-inflammatory properties
Lupeol	Olive, mango, strawberries, grapes, figs, many vegetables and medicinal plants	Antioxidant, anti-inflammatory, anti-mutagenic, inhibits the activity of DNA topoisomerase II, a target for anticancer chemotherapy
Terpenoids		
Bilobalide and ginkgolide	Ginkgo leaves	Antioxidant, antilipoperoxidative properties, apoptosis of cancer cells

resources

Throughout the book, Step by Step, we give you references (a) to substantiate the points we are making and (b) to enable you or your health professionals to dig into the relevant literature further. Here, we give you a series of resources to help you find more details of the various topics covered in the book and find help, for example from charities. Two kinds of resource are given: books and websites. All the recommended books have been read by us and their contents are reliable. However, books can become outdated quickly, especially in a fast-moving field like cancer, whereas websites can readily and regularly be updated. Also, do remember our advice regarding websites (page 86). The resources listed are generally meant to give you a flavour of what kind of literature to look for. The list is by no means exhaustive.

books

Mukherjee, Siddhartha (2011) *The Emperor of All Maladies*. HarperCollins.

Rosenberg, Steven A. and Barry, John M. (1992) *The Transformed Cell*. Phoenix.

Skloot, Rebecca (2010) *The Immortal Life of Henrietta Lacks*. Pan Books.

Pecorino, Lauren (2011) *Why Millions Survive Cancer*. Oxford University Press.

Scientific American (Special Edition) – *New Answers for Cancer* (2008).

Weinberg, Robert A. (2013) *The Biology of Cancer*. 2nd Ed. Garland Science.

Alberts, Bruce, Johnson, Alexander, Lewis, Julian, Raff, Martin, Roberts, Keith and Walter, Peter (2008) *Molecular Biology of the Cell.* 5th Ed. Garland Science.

Hasketh, Robin (2013) *Introduction to Cancer Biology.* Cambridge University Press.

Abrams, Donald and Weil, Andrew (2009) *Integrative Oncology.* Oxford University Press.

Campbell, C. T. and Campbell, T. M. (2006) *The China Study: the most comprehensive study of nutrition ever conducted and the startling implications for diet, weight loss and long-term health.* BenBella Books.

Carey, Nessa (2011) *The Epigenetics Revolution: How Modern Biology is Rewriting Our Understanding of Genetics, Disease and Inheritance.* Icon Books.

Plant, Jane (2007) *Your Life in Your Hands.* Fourth edition. Virgin Books.

Plant, Jane (2007) *Understand, prevent and overcome prostate cancer.* Revised edition. Virgin Books.

Plant, Jane and Stephenson, Janet (2011) *Beating Stress, Anxiety and Depression.* Reprint edition. Piatkus.

Plant, Jane and Tidey, Gill (2004) *The Plant Programme.* Revised edition. Virgin Books.

Plant, Jane, Tidey, Gill (2010) *Eating for Better Health.* Virgin Books.

Plant, J. A., Voulvoulis, Nikolaos and Ragnarsdottir, Vala (editors) (2012) *Pollutants, human health and the environment: a risk based approach.* Wiley-Blackwell, London.

websites

National Health Service – Cancer (NHS Choices) – http://www.nhs.uk/cancer

American Cancer Society – http://www.cancer.org

World Health Organization (WHO) – http://www.who.int

Mayo Clinic – http://www.mayoclinic.org

Memorial Sloan-Kettering Cancer Center – http://www.mskcc.org

MD Anderson Cancer Center – www.mdanderson.org

Cancer Research UK – http://www.cancerresearchuk.org

American Association for Cancer Research (AACR) – http://www.aacr.org

Macmillan Cancer Support – http://www.macmillan.org.uk

National Cancer Institute – www.cancer.gov

http://www.naturalnews.com/033694_chemicals_cosmetics.html#ixzz20PihCdBs

http://www.mayoclinic.com/health/cancer/DS01076

http://www.cancercenter.com/after-care-services/protein.cfm

http://www.cancer.gov/cancertopics/coping/life-after-treatment/page1/AllPages

http://www.macmillan.org.uk/Cancerinformation/Livingwithandaftercancer/Lifeaftercancer/Lifeaftercancer.aspx

http://www.walkingforhealth.org.uk

Gaia House http://gaiahouse.co.uk/

For Sangha groups see http://gaiahouse.co.uk/local-meditation-groups/

The Community of Interbeing UK http://www.coiuk.org/ For groups see http://www.coiuk.org/local-groups/find-a-local-group/

acknowledgements

The authors received help and support from many friends and colleagues. They would like in particular to thank Pat Goodall and Anne Montague, two excellent journalists who helped ensure the book was written in accessible English. Dr Scott Fraser helped with library research and referencing and Dr Mine Guzel prepared the diagrams. Dr Henry Haslam helped with the final editing. We thank them all very much.

We also thank our reviewers who read one or more chapters and made helpful and constructive comments. They included in alphabetical order Dr Michael Dixon, Lynn Faulds Wood, Professor Stephen Holgate CBE, Dr Christian Ihlenfeld, Dr Michael Mcintyre, Professor Alexander Orlov, Dr Robert Owen, Dr Tej Samani, Jo Sawicki, Professor Michael Seckl, Dr Thomas Simpson, Elodie Stanley, Professor Justin Stebbing, Dr Siegfried Trefzer, Dr Maria Vlachopoulou and Dr Nick Voulvoulis. A particularly generous financial donation was received from The Stanley Foundation Ltd.

We are grateful to Susanna Abbott, publishing director at Vermilion Books, for commissioning the book and helping to shape it, to Catherine Knight, assistant editor at Vermilion, for help with the manuscript and proofs and Toby Clarke, who designed the book cover.

Mustafa wishes to thank his wife Sabire and Jane thanks her husband Professor Peter Simpson for their constant help and support.

endnotes

Welcome

1. www.cancerresearchuk.org/
2. Plant, J.A., Bone, J., Kinniburgh, D.G., Smedley, P.L., Fordyce, F.M., Klinck, B.A. and Voulvoulis, N., 2013. Arsenic and Selenium. In: *Treatise on Geochemistry*, 2nd Ed (editors H.D. Holland and K.K. Turekian). Elsevier, Oxford.
3. Plant, J. A., Voulvoulis, Nikolaos and Ragnarsdottir, Vala (editors), 2012. *Pollutants, human health and the environment: a risk based approach.* Wiley-Blackwell, London.
4. Plant, Jane, 2000. *Your Life in Your Hands.* Virgin Books; now in its fourth edition, 2007.
5. Plant, Jane and Tidey, Gill, 2001. *The Plant Programme.* Virgin Books; revised edition 2004.
6. Plant, Jane, 2007. *Your Life in Your Hands.* Fourth edition. Virgin Books; Plant, Jane and Tidey, Gill, 2004. *The Plant Programme.* Revised edition. Virgin Books; Plant, Jane, 2007. *Understand, prevent and overcome prostate cancer.* Revised edition. Virgin Books.
7. Cancer Research UK, 2010.

Step 1

1. Masson, S., Bahl, A. (2012) Metastatic castrate-resistant prostate cancer: dawn of a new age of management. *British Journal of Urology International*, 110 (8), 1110-1114.
2. http://www.macmillan.org.uk/Cancerinformation/Aboutcancer/Whogets cancer.aspx
3. http://cancerhelp.cancerresearchuk.org/about-cancer/cancer-questions/ childrens-cancers
4. Popkin, B.M. (2007) Science and society – Understanding global nutrition dynamics as a step towards controlling cancer incidence. *Nature Reviews Cancer*, 7 (1), 61-67.
5. http://www.who.int/en/
6. Plant, Jane, 2007. *Your Life in Your Hands.* Fourth edition. Virgin Books.
7. Hanahan, D., Weinberg, R.A. (2000) The hallmarks of cancer. *Cell*, 100 (1), 57-70.
8. Hanahan, D., Weinberg, R.A. (2011) Hallmarks of cancer: The next generation. *Cell*, 144 (5), 646-674.
9. Greenwald P (2002) Cancer chemoprevention. *BMJ.* 2002 Mar 23;324(7339): 714-8.
10. Campbell, C. T., Campbell, T. M. (2006) *The China Study: the most comprehensive study of nutrition ever conducted and the starting implications for diet, weight loss and long-term health.* Dallas, Texas. BenBella Books.
11. Plant, Jane, 2007. *Your Life in Your Hands.* Fourth edition. Virgin Books.

12 Holmgren. L., O'Reilly, M.S., Folkman, J. (1995) Dormancy of micrometastases: balanced proliferation and apoptosis in the presence of angiogenesis suppression. *Nature Medicine*, 1 (2), 149–53.

13 Stafford, L.J., Vaidya, K.S., Welch, D.R. (2008) Metastasis suppressors genes in cancer. *International Journal Of Biochemistry & Cell Biology*, 40 (5), 874-891.

14 http://dx.doi.org/10.1038/nature12968

15 http://www.nature.com/news/cancer-stem-cells-tracked-1.11087

16 International Human Genome Sequencing Consortium (2004). Finishing the euchromatic sequence of the human genome. *Nature*, 431 (7011), 931–945.

17 Colbourne, J.K., Pfrender, M.E., Gilbert, D., Thomas, W.K., Tucker, A., Oakley, T.H., et al., (2011). The ecoresponsive genome of *Daphnia pulex*. *Science*, 331 (6017), 555-561.

18 Carey, Nessa (2011) *The Epigenetics Revolution: How Modern Biology is Rewriting Our Understanding of Genetics, Disease and Inheritance*. Icon Books.

19 Plant, Jane, 2007. *Your Life in Your Hands*. Fourth edition. Virgin Books.

20 Carey, Nessa (2011) *The Epigenetics Revolution: How Modern Biology is Rewriting Our Understanding of Genetics, Disease and Inheritance*. Icon Books; and references therein.

21 McGowan et al (2008) Diet and the epigenetic (re)programming of phenotypic differences in behaviour. *Brain Res.*, 1237: 1224; Nyström et al (2009) Diet and epigenetics in colon cancer. *World J Gastroenterol.* 2009 January 21; 15(3): 257 263).

22 Kronenwetter C, Weidner G, Pettengill E, Marlin R, Crutchfield L, McCormac P, Raisin CJ, Ornish DA (2005) A qualitative analysis of interviews of men with early stage prostate cancer: the Prostate Cancer Lifestyle Trial. *Cancer Nurs.* 2005 Mar-Apr;28(2):99-107.

23 Ornish, D., Magbanua, M.J.M., Weidner, G., Weinberg, V., Kemp, C., Green, C., et al. (2008) Changes in prostate gene expression in men undergoing an intensive nutrition and lifestyle intervention. *Proceedings of the National Academy of Sciences of the United States of America*, 105 (24), 8369-8374.

24 Onkal, R., Djamgoz, M.B.A. (2009) Molecular pharmacology of voltage-gated sodium channel expression in metastatic disease: Clinical potential of neonatal Nav1.5 in breast cancer. *European Journal of Pharmacology*, 25 December 2009, 206–219; Djamgoz, M.B.A., Onkal, R. (2013) Persistent current blockers of voltage-gated sodium channels: A clinical opportunity for controlling metastatic disease. *Recent Patents on Anti-Cancer Drug Discovery*, 8 (1), 66-84.

25 Djamgoz, M.B.A. (2011) Bioelectricity of Cancer, in *The Physiology of Bioelectricity in Development, Tissue Regeneration and Cancer*. Ed., Pullar C.E., CRC Press, UK. Pp 269-294.

26 House, C.D., Vaske, C.J., Schwartz, A.M., Obias, V., Frank, B., Luu, T. et al. (2010) Voltage-gated Na+ channel SCN5A is a key regulator of a gene transcriptional network that controls colon cancer invasion. *Cancer Research*, 70 (17), 6957-6567.

27 Fraser SP, Ozerlat-Gunduz I, Brackenbury WJ, Fitzgerald EM, Campbell TM, Coombes RC, Djamgoz MB. Regulation of voltage-gated sodium channel expression in cancer: hormones, growth factors and auto-regulation. Philos Trans R Soc Lond B Biol Sci. 2014 Feb 3;369(1638):20130105. doi: 10.1098/rstb.2013.0105.

Brackenbury WJ and Djamgoz MBA (2007) Nerve growth factor enhances voltage-gated Na+ channel activity and Transwell migration in Mat-LyLu rat prostate cancer cell line. *Journal of Cellular Physiology*, 210: 602-608; Uysal-

Onganer P and Djamgoz MBA (2007) Epidermal growth factor potentiates in vitro metastatic behaviour of human prostate cancer PC-3M cells: involvement of voltage-gated sodium channel. *Molecular Cancer* 6: 7; Ding Y, Brackenbury WJ, Onganer PU, Montano X, Porter LM, Bates LF, Djamgoz MBA (2008) Epidermal growth factor upregulates motility of Mat-LyLu rat prostate cancer cells partially via voltage-gated Na+ channel activity. *Journal of Cellular Physiology*, 215: 77-81; Fraser SP, Ozerlat-Gunduz I, Onkal R, Diss JK, Latchman DS and Djamgoz MB (2010) Estrogen and non-genomic upregulation of voltage-gated Na(+) channel activity in MDA-MB-231 human breast cancer cells: role in adhesion. *J Cell Physiol*, 224: 527-539; Tabb, J.S., Fanger, G.R., Wilson, E.M., Maue, R.A., Henderson, L.P. (1994) Suppression of sodium channel function in differentiating C2 muscle cells stably overexpressing rat androgen receptors. *Journal of Neuroscience* 14 (2), 763-773; Zakon, H.H. (1998). The effects of steroid hormones on electrical activity of excitable cells. *Trends in Neurosciences*, 21 (5), 202-207.

28 Wallace CHR, Baczkó I, Jones L, Fercho M and Light PE (2006) Inhibition of cardiac voltage-gated sodium channels by grape polyphenols. *Br J Pharmacol*, 149: 657-665; Isbilen B, Fraser SP and Djamgoz MB (2006) Docosahexaenoic acid (omega-3) blocks voltage-gated sodium channel activity and migration of MDA-MB-231 human breast cancer cells. *Int J Biochem Cell Biol*, 38: 2173-2182; T Nakajima, N Kubota, T Tsutsumi, A Oguri, H Imuta, T Jo, H Oonuma, M Soma, K Meguro, H Takano, T Nagase, and T Nagata (2009) Eicosapentaenoic acid inhibits voltage-gated sodium channels and invasiveness in prostate cancer cells. *Br J Pharmacol*, 156: 420-431; Liu L, Oortgiesen M, Li L and Simon SA (2001) Capsaicin inhibits activation of voltage-gated sodium currents in capsaicin-sensitive trigeminal ganglion neurons. *J Neurophysiol*, 85: 745-758; Deng HM, Yin ST, Yan D, Tang ML, Li CC, Chen JT, Wang M & Ruan DY (2008) Effects of EGCG on voltage-gated sodium channels in primary cultures of rat hippocampal CA1 neurons. *Toxicology*, 252: 1-8.

29 Djamgoz, M.B.A., Onkal, R. (2013) Persistent current blockers of voltage-gated sodium channels: A clinical opportunity for controlling metastatic disease. *Recent Patents on Anti-Cancer Drug Discovery*, 8 (1), 66-84.

30 Kim, J. and Dang, C (2006) Cancer's Molecular Sweet Tooth and the Warburg Effect. *Cancer Res* September 15, 2006 66; 8927.

31 Zhang, X., Tworoger, S.S., Eliassen, A.H., Hankinson, S.E. (2013) Postmenopausal plasma sex hormone levels and breast cancer risk over 20 years of follow-up. *Breast Cancer Research and Treatment*. 137 (3), 883-892.

32 Jaakkola S, Lyytinen HK, Pukkala E, Ylikorkala O. (2011) Use of estradiol-progestin therapy associates with increased risk for uterine sarcomas. *Gynecol Oncol*. 2011 Aug;122(2):260-3. doi: 10.1016/j.ygyno.2011.04.003. Epub 2011 Apr 30.

33 http://monographs.iarc.fr/ENG/Monographs/vol72/mono72-8.pdf

34 Chaves J, Saif MW (2011) IGF system in cancer: from bench to clinic. *Anticancer Drugs*. 2011 Mar;22(3):206-12; Chen, W., Wang, S., Tian, T., Bai, J.L., Hu, Z.B., Xu, Y. et al. (2009) Phenotypes and genotypes of insulin-like growth factor 1 IGF-binding protein-3 and cancer risk: evidence from 96 studies. *European Journal of Human Genetics*, 17 (12) 1668-1675.

35 Tata JR (1996) Metamorphosis: an exquisite model for hormonal regulation of post-embryonic development. *Biochem Soc Symp*. 1996;62:123-36.

36 Alberts B, Johnson A, Lewis J, et al. (2002) *Molecular Biology of the Cell*. 4th edition. New York: Garland Science.

37   Kleinberg, D.L. (1998) Role of IGF-1 in normal mammary development. *Breast Cancer Research and Treatment*, 47 (3), 201-208; Perry, R.J., Farquharson, C., Ahmed, S.F. (2008) The role of sex steroids in controlling pubertal growth. *Clinical Endocrinology*, 68 (1), 4-15.

38   e.g. Chi F, Wu R, Zeng YC, Xing R, Liu Y (2012) Circulation insulin-like growth factor peptides and colorectal cancer risk: an updated systematic review and meta-analysis. *Mol Biol Rep*. 2012 Dec 27. [Epub ahead of print.]

39   Wehland, M., Bauer, J., Infanger, M., Grimm, D. (2012) Target-based anti-angiogenic therapy in breast cancer. *Current Pharmaceutical Design*, 18 (27) 4244-4257.

40   Wehland, M., Bauer, J., Infanger, M., Grimm, D. (2012) Target-based anti-angiogenic therapy in breast cancer. *Current Pharmaceutical Design*, 18 (27) 4244-4257.

Step 2 Find Your Balance

1   Beales, D. (2004) Beyond mind-body dualism: implications for patient care. *Journal of Holistic Healthcare*, 1 (3), 15-22.

2   Guyton, A. L., Hall, J. E. (2001) *Textbook of medical physiology* [10th Edition. Philadelphia.]

3   Murrell, A., Uribe-Lewis, S. (2012) Genomic imprinting and cancer. *Biochemist*, 32 (5), 26-29.

4   Servan-Schreiber, D. (2005) *Healing without Freud or Prozac: Natural approaches to curing stress, anxiety and depression.* [Revised edition.] London, Rodale Publishing Ltd.

5   Maclean, P. (1990) *The triune brain in evolution: Role of paleocerebral functions.* USA, Plenum Press.

6   Ornish, D.M., Magbanua, M. J. M., Weidner, G., Weinberg, V., Kemp, C., Green, C., Mattie, M., Marlin, R., Simko, J., Shinohara, K., Haqq, C. M., Carroll, P. R. (2008) Changes in prostate gene expression in men undergoing an intensive nutrition and lifestyle intervention. *Proceedings of the National Academy of Sciences*, 105 (24), 8369-8374.

Step 3 Choosing the Right Conventional Therapies for You

1   Sasieni PD, Shelton J, Ormiston-Smith N, Thomson CS & Silcocks PB (2011) What is the lifetime risk of developing cancer?: The effect of adjusting for multiple primaries. *Br J Cancer*, 105: 460-465.

2   Walters S, Maringe C, Butler J, Rachet B, Barrett-Lee P, Bergh J, Boyages J, Christiansen P, Lee M, Wärnberg F, Allemani C, Engholm G, Fornander T, Gjerstorff ML, Johannesen TB, Lawrence G, McGahan CE, Middleton R, Steward J, Tracey E, Turner D, Richards MA, Coleman MP (2013) Breast cancer survival and stage at diagnosis in Australia, Canada, Denmark, Norway, Sweden and the UK, 2000-2007: a population-based study. *Br J Cancer*. [Epub ahead of print.]

3   http://www.breakthrough.org.uk/media_centre/news_views/breast_cancer_4.html

4   http://www.cancerscreening.nhs.uk/bowel/publications/colonoscopy-investigation.pdf

5   http://www.cancerresearchuk.org/cancer-info/spotcancerearly/key-signs-and-symptoms/

6   http://www.bbc.co.uk/news/health-19662456

7   http://www.telegraph.co.uk/health/healthnews/9438046

8   Bleyer, Archie and H. Gilbert Welch (2012). Effect of Three Decades of Screening

Mammography on Breast-Cancer Incidence. *N Engl J Med*; 367:1998-2005. November 22, 2012.

9   Marmot MG, Altman DG, Cameron DA, Dewar JA, Thompson SG, Wilcox M. Independent UK Panel on Breast Cancer Screening. The benefits and harms of breast cancer screening: an independent review. *Lancet*. 2012 Nov 17;380(9855):1778-86.

10   Marmot MG, Altman DG, Cameron DA, Dewar JA, Thompson SG, Wilcox M. Independent UK Panel on Breast Cancer Screening. The benefits and harms of breast cancer screening: an independent review. *Lancet*. 2012 Nov 17;380(9855):1778-86.

11   http://www.cancerscreening.nhs.uk/bowel/publications/bowel-cancer-the-facts. pdf

12   Hewitson P, Glasziou PP, Irwig L, Towler B, Watson E. (2007) Screening for colorectal cancer using the faecal occult blood test, Hemoccult. *Cochrane Database of Systematic Reviews 2007*, Issue 1. Art. No.: CD001216.

13   Peto J, Gilham C, Fletcher O, Matthews FE (2004) The cervical cancer epidemic that screening has prevented in the UK. *Lancet*. 2004 Jul 17-23;364(9430):249-56; Bryant E (2012) The impact of policy and screening on cervical cancer in England. *Br J Nurs*. 2012 Feb 23-Mar 7;21(4):S4, S6-10.

14   http://www.ons.gov.uk/ons/index.html

15   http://www.cancer.org/cancer/prostatecancer/detailedguide/prostate-cancer-key-statistics

16   Jemal A, Siegel R, Ward E et al. (2006) Cancer statistics, 2006. *CA Cancer J Clin* 2006 Mar-Apr;56(2):106–130.

17   Ilic D, Neuberger MM, Djulbegovic M, Dahm P. (2013) Screening for prostate cancer. *Cochrane Database Syst Rev*. 2013 Jan 31;1:CD004720.

18   Ilic D, Neuberger MM, Djulbegovic M, Dahm P. (2013) Screening for prostate cancer. *Cochrane Database Syst Rev*. 2013 Jan 31;1:CD004720.

19   Klotz L (2012) Active surveillance for favorable-risk prostate cancer: background, patient selection, triggers for intervention, and outcomes. *Curr Urol Rep*. 2012 Apr;13(2):153-9. doi: 10.1007/s11934-012-0242-4.

20   Shah DJ, Sachs RK, Wilson DJ (2012) Radiation-induced cancer: a modern view. *Br J Radiol*. 2012 Dec;85(1020):e1166-73.

21   http://www.cancerresearchuk.org/cancer-help/about-cancer/tests/ultrasound-scan

22   http://www.cancerresearchuk.org/cancer-help/about-cancer/tests/mri-scan

23   http://www.cancerresearchuk.org/cancer-help/about-cancer/tests/pet-scan

24   http://www.cancerresearchuk.org/cancer-help/about-cancer/tests/petct-scan

25   Nievelstein RA, Quarles van Ufford HM, Kwee TC, Bierings MB, Ludwig I, Beek FJ, de Klerk JM, Mali WP, de Bruin PW, Geleijns (2012) Radiation exposure and mortality risk from CT and PET imaging of patients with malignant lymphoma. *J. Eur Radiol*. 2012 Sep;22(9):1946-54.

26   http://www.cancerresearchuk.org/cancer-help/about-cancer/tests/blood-tests

27   http://www.cancerresearchuk.org/cancer-help/about-cancer/cancer-questions/what-is-a-normal-full-blood-count

28   Fine JH, Chen P, Mesci A, Allan DS, Gasser S, Raulet DH, Carlyle JR. (2010) Chemotherapy-induced genotoxic stress promotes sensitivity to natural killer cell cytotoxicity by enabling missing-self recognition. *Cancer Res*. 2010 Sep 15;70(18):7102-13.

29   http://www.cancerresearchuk.org/cancer-help/about-cancer/cancer-questions/liver-function-tests

30 Neville AM, Mackay AM, Westwood J, Turberville C, Laurence DJ (1975) Human tumour-associated and tumour-specific antigens: some concepts in relation to clinical oncology. *J Clin Pathol Suppl (Assoc Clin Pathol)*. 1975;6: 102-12.

31 Parkinson DR, Dracopoli N, Petty BG, Compton C, Cristofanilli M, Deisseroth A, Hayes DF, Kapke G, Kumar P, Lee JSh, Liu MC, McCormack R, Mikulski S, Nagahara L, Pantel K, Pearson-White S, Punnoose EA, Roadcap LT, Schade AE, Scher HI, Sigman CC, Kelloff GJ. (2012) Considerations in the development of circulating tumor cell technology for clinical use. *J Transl Med*. 2012 Jul 2;10:138. doi: 10.1186/1479-5876-10-138.

32 http://www.genome.gov/10000533

33 Sanoudou D, Mountzios G, Arvanitis DA, Pectasides D. (2012) Array-based pharmacogenomics of molecular-targeted therapies in oncology. *Pharmacogenomics J*. 2012 Jun;12(3):185-96.

34 Amiel J, de Pontual L, Henrion-Caude A. (2012) miRNA, development and disease. *Adv Genet*. 2012;80:1-36.

35 Nana-Sinkam SP, Croce CM. (2013) Clinical applications for microRNAs in cancer. *Clin Pharmacol Ther*. 2013 Jan;93(1):98-104.

36 Lindon JC, Holmes E, Nicholson JK (2004) Metabonomics: systems biology in pharmaceutical research and development. *Curr Opin Mol Ther*. 2004 Jun;6(3):265-72.

37 Claudino WM, Goncalves PH, di Leo A, Philip PA, Sarkar FH (2012) Metabolomics in cancer: a bench-to-bedside intersection. *Crit Rev Oncol Hematol*. 2012 Oct;84(1):1-7. doi: 10.1016/j.critrevonc.2012.02.009. Epub 2012 Mar 18.

38 http://www.cancer.gov/cancertopics/genetics/breast/predictive-testing-p53-mutations

39 Urquidi V, Rosser CJ, Goodison S. (2012) Molecular diagnostic trends in urological cancer: Biomarkers for non-invasive diagnosis. *Curr Med Chem*. 2012;19(22):3653-63

40 http://www.cancerresearchuk.org/cancer-help/utilities/glossary/urea-and-electrolytes

41 Sriram KB, Relan V, Clarke BE, Duhig EE, Yang IA, Bowman RV, Lee YC, Fong KM. (2011) Diagnostic molecular biomarkers for malignant pleural effusions. *Future Oncol*. 2011 Jun;7(6):737-52.

42 http://www.cancer.gov/cancertopics/factsheet/detection/tumor-grade

43 http://www.nhs.uk/conditions/Mastectomy/Pages/Introduction.aspx

44 Sarder P, Gullicksrud K, Mondal S, Sudlow GP, Achilefu S, Akers WJ. (2013) Dynamic optical projection of acquired luminescence for aiding oncologic surgery. *J Biomed Opt*. 2013 Dec 1;18(12):120501. doi: 10.1117/1. JBO.18.12.120501.

45 Ghiaur G, Gerber J, Jones RJ (2012) Concise review: Cancer stem cells and minimal residual disease. *Stem Cells*. 2012 Jan;30(1):89-93.

46 Gieni M, Avram R, Dickson L, Farrokhyar F, Lovrics P, Faidi S, Sne N. (2012) Local breast cancer recurrence after mastectomy and immediate breast reconstruction for invasive cancer: a meta-analysis. *Breast*. 2012 Jun;21(3):230-6.

47 http://www.cancer.gov/cancertopics/factsheet/Therapy/cryosurgery

48 Tremp M, Hefermehl L, Largo R, Knönagel H, Sulser T, Eberli D. (2011) Electrosurgery in urology: recent advances. *Expert Rev Med Devices*. 2011 Sep;8(5):597-605; Kim JH, Park JY, Kim DY, Kim YM, Kim YT, Nam JH (2009) The role of loop electrosurgical excisional procedure in the management

of adenocarcinoma in situ of the uterine cervix. *Eur J Obstet Gynecol Reprod Biol.* 2009 Jul;145(1):100-3.

49 Olson JM, Alam M, Asgari MM. (2012) Needs assessment for general dermatologic surgery. *Dermatol Clin.* 2012 Jan;30(1):153-66.

50 http://www.nhs.uk/conditions/Laparoscopy/Pages/Introduction.aspx

51 Franceschini G, Terribile D, Magno S, Fabbri C, Accetta C, Di Leone A, Moschella F, Barbarino R, Scaldaferri A, Darchi S, Carvelli ME, Bove S, Masetti R (2012) Update on oncoplastic breast surgery. *Eur Rev Med Pharmacol Sci.* 2012 Oct;16(11):1530-40.

52 Mitchell OR (2012) Current advances in facial reconstructive surgery following head and neck cancer surgery. *Plast Surg Nurs.* 2012 Jan-Mar;32(1):6-9; quiz 10-1. doi: 10.1097/PSN.0b013e318244f9f0.

53 http://www.cancerresearchuk.org/cancer-help/about-cancer/treatment/chemotherapy

54 Humphrey Rachel W, Brockway-Lunardi Laura M, Bonk David T, Dohoney Kathleen M, Doroshow James H, Meech Sandra J, Ratain Mark J, Topalian Suzanne L, and Pardoll Drew M (2011) Opportunities and Challenges in the Development of Experimental Drug Combinations for Cancer. *J. Natl. Cancer Inst.* 2011 103: 1222-1226.

55 http://www.cancerresearchuk.org/cancer-help/type/bladder-cancer/treatment/early/treatment-into-the-bladder#chemo

56 Lacarrubba F, Potenza MC, Gurgone S, Micali G. (2011) Successful treatment and management of large superficial basal cell carcinomas with topical imiquimod 5% cream: a case series and review. *J Dermatolog Treat.* 2011 Dec;22(6):353-8.

57 http://www.cancerresearchuk.org/cancer-help/about-cancer/treatment/chemotherapy/plan

58 http://www.cancerresearchuk.org/cancer-help/about-cancer/treatment/chemotherapy/chemotherapy-side-effects

59 e.g. Mengyuan Du, Xujuan Yang, James A. Hartman, Paul S. Cooke, Daniel R. Doerge, Young H. Ju, and William G. Helferich. (2012) Low-dose dietary genistein negates the therapeutic effect of tamoxifen in athymic nude mice. *Carcinogenesis* 2012 33: 895-901.

60 http://www.macmillan.org.uk/Cancerinformation/Cancertreatment/Treatmenttypes/Chemotherapy/Linesports/PICCline.aspx

61 http://www.macmillan.org.uk/Cancerinformation/Cancertreatment/Treatmenttypes/Chemotherapy/Linesports/Implantableport.aspx

62 http://www.cancerresearchuk.org/cancer-help/about-cancer/treatment/chemotherapy/having/chemotherapy-pumps

63 Schnell FM (2003) Chemotherapy-induced nausea and vomiting: the importance of acute antiemetic control. *Oncologist.* 2003;8(2):187-98.

64 e.g. Cohen, Adam D., Kemeny Nancy E. (2003) An Update on Hepatic Arterial Infusion Chemotherapy for Colorectal Cancer. *The Oncologist* 2003; 8:553-566; Masanori Nakanishia, Yukihiro Umedaa, Yoshiki Demuraa, Shingo Ameshimaa, Yukio Chibab, Isamu Miyamoria, Takeshi Ishizakic. (2007) Effective use of multi-arterial infusion chemotherapy for advanced non-small cell lung cancer patients: Four clinical specified cases. *Lung Cancer* 55, 2, February 2007, 241–247; Love, Susan M., Wei Zhang, Eva J. Gordon, Jianyu Rao, Hongying Yang, Junyao Li, Bailin Zhang, Xiang Wang, Guoji Chen, and Baoning Zhang (2013) A Feasibility Study of the Intraductal Administration of Chemotherapy. *Cancer Prev Res* January 2013 6:51-58.

65 Singh S, Sharma A, Robertson GP (2012) Realizing the clinical potential of cancer nanotechnology by minimizing toxicologic and targeted delivery concerns. *Cancer Res.* 2012 Nov 15;72(22):5663-8.

66 Mali B, Jarm T, Snoj M, Sersa G, Miklavcic D (2013) Antitumor effectiveness of electrochemotherapy: a systematic review and meta-analysis. *Eur J Surg Oncol.* 2013 Jan;39(1):4-16.

67 Baskar R, Lee KA, Yeo R, Yeoh KW. (2012) Cancer and radiation therapy: current advances and future directions. *Int J Med Sci.* 2012;9(3):193-9.

68 Ibid. Baskar R, Lee KA, Yeo R, Yeoh KW. (2012) Cancer and Radiation Therapy: Current Advances and Future Directions. *Int J Med Sci*; 9(3):193-199.

69 Lo SS, Fakiris AJ, Chang EL, Mayr NA, Wang JZ, Papiez L, Teh BS, McGarry RC, Cardenes HR, Timmerman RD. (2010) Stereotactic body radiation therapy: a novel treatment modality. *Nat Rev Clin Oncol.* 2010 Jan;7(1):44-54. Erratum in: *Nat Rev Clin Oncol.* 2010 Aug;7(8):422.

70 Jaffray D, Kupelian P, Djemil T, Macklis RM (2007) Review of image-guided radiation therapy. *Expert Rev Anticancer Ther.* 2007 Jan;7(1):89-103.

71 Sfoungaristos S, Giannitsas K, Perimenis P (2011) Present and future therapeutic options for locally advanced and metastatic renal cell carcinoma. *Expert Opin Pharmacother.* 2011 Mar;12(4):533-47; Pak BJ, Lee J, Thai BL, Fuchs SY, Shaked Y, Ronai Z, Kerbel RS, Ben-David Y. (2004) Radiation resistance of human melanoma analysed by retroviral insertional mutagenesis reveals a possible role for dopachrome tautomerase. *Oncogene.* 2004 Jan 8;23(1):30-8; Moncharmont C, Levy A, Gilormini M, Bertrand G, Chargari C, Alphonse G, Ardail D, Rodriguez-Lafrasse C, Magné N (2012) Targeting a cornerstone of radiation resistance: cancer stem cell. *Cancer Lett.* 2012 Sep 28;322(2):139-47.

72 Dumont F, Altmeyer A, Bischoff P. (2009) Radiosensitising agents for the radiotherapy of cancer: novel molecularly targeted approaches. *Expert Opin Ther Pat.* 2009 Jun;19(6):775-99; Bischoff P, Altmeyer A, Dumont F. (2009) Radiosensitising agents for the radiotherapy of cancer: advances in traditional and hypoxia targeted radiosensitisers. *Expert Opin Ther Pat.* 2009 May;19(5): 643-62.

73 Al-Bataineh O, Jenne J, Huber P (2012) Clinical and future applications of high intensity focused ultrasound in cancer. *Cancer Treat Rev.* 2012 Aug;38(5): 346-53.

74 Li C, Zhang W, Fan W, Huang J, Zhang F, Wu P (2010) Noninvasive treatment of malignant bone tumors using high-intensity focused ultrasound. *Cancer.* 2010 Aug 15;116(16):3934-42; Khokhlova TD, Hwang JH (2011) HIFU for palliative treatment of pancreatic cancer. *J Gastrointest Oncol.* 2011 Sep;2(3): 175-84.

75 Grüll H, Langereis S (2012) Hyperthermia-triggered drug delivery from temperature-sensitive liposomes using MRI-guided high intensity focused ultrasound. *J Control Release.* 2012 Jul 20;161(2):317-27.

76 Levivier M, Gevaert T, Negretti L (2011) Gamma Knife, CyberKnife, Tomo Therapy: gadgets or useful tools? *Curr Opin Neurol.* 2011 Dec;24(6):616-25.

77 Haie-Meder C, Siebert FA, Pötter R. Image guided, adaptive, accelerated, high dose brachytherapy as model for advanced small volume radiotherapy. *Radiother Oncol.* 2011 Sep;100(3):333-43.

78 Ovarian ablation for early breast cancer. Early Breast Cancer Trialists' Collaborative Group. *Cochrane Database Syst Rev.* 2000;(3):CD000485.

79 Turkistani A, Marsh S. (2012) Pharmacogenomics of third-generation aromatase inhibitors. *Expert Opin Pharmacother.* 2012 Jun;13(9):1299-307.

80 Ali S, Buluwela L, Coombes RC. (2011) Antiestrogens and their therapeutic applications in breast cancer and other diseases. *Annu Rev Med.* 2011;62:217-32; Ko SS, Jordan VC. (2011) Treatment of osteoporosis and reduction in risk

of invasive breast cancer in postmenopausal women with raloxifene. *Expert Opin Pharmacother*. 2011 Mar;12(4):657-74.

81 Hayes E, Nicholson RI, Hiscox S. (2011) Acquired endocrine resistance in breast cancer: implications for tumour metastasis. *Front Biosci*. 2011 Jan 1;16:838-48; Tombal B. (2011) What is the pathophysiology of a hormone-resistant prostate tumour? *Eur J Cancer*. 2011 Sep;47 Suppl 3:S179-88.

82 Bauer K, Rancea M, Roloff V, Elter T, Hallek M, Engert A, Skoetz N (2012) Rituximab, ofatumumab and other monoclonal anti-CD20 antibodies for chronic lymphocytic leukaemia. *Cochrane Database Syst Rev*. 2012 Nov 14;11:CD008079.

83 Wilson PM, LaBonte MJ, Lenz HJ. (2013) Assessing the in vivo efficacy of biologic antiangiogenic therapies. *Cancer Chemother Pharmacol*. 2013 Jan;71(1):1-12; Wu JM, Staton CA (2012) Anti-angiogenic drug discovery: lessons from the past and thoughts for the future. *Expert Opin Drug Discov*. 2012 Aug;7(8):723-43; Braghiroli MI, Sabbaga J, Hoff PM. (2012) Bevacizumab: overview of the literature. *Expert Rev Anticancer Ther*. 2012 May;12(5):567-80.

84 Moja L, Tagliabue L, Balduzzi S, Parmelli E, Pistotti V, Guarneri V, D'Amico R. (2012) Trastuzumab containing regimens for early breast cancer. *Cochrane Database Syst Rev*. 2012 Apr 18;4:CD006243; Smyth EC, Cunningham D. (2012) Targeted therapy for gastric cancer. *Curr Treat Options Oncol*. 2012 Sep;13(3):377-89.

85 Melief CJ, O'Shea JJ, Stroncek DF. (2011) Summit on cell therapy for cancer: The importance of the interaction of multiple disciplines to advance clinical therapy. *J Transl Med*. 2011 Jul 8;9:107; Koh MB, Suck G. (2012) Cell therapy: promise fulfilled? *Biologicals*. 2012 May;40(3):214-7.

86 Akao Y, Ebihara T, Masuda H, Saeki Y, Akazawa T, Hazeki K, Hazeki O, Matsumoto M, Seya T. (2009) Enhancement of antitumor natural killer cell activation by orally administered Spirulina extract in mice. *Cancer Sci*. 2009 Aug;100(8):1494-501.

87 Kim BK, Han KH, Ahn SH. (2011) Prevention of hepatocellular carcinoma in patients with chronic hepatitis B virus infection. *Oncology*. 2011;81 Suppl 1: 41-9.

88 Gardner TA, Elzey BD, Hahn NM. (2012) Sipuleucel-T (Provenge) autologous vaccine approved for treatment of men with asymptomatic or minimally symptomatic castrate-resistant metastatic prostate cancer. *Hum Vaccin Immunother*. 2012 Apr;8(4):534-9.

89 Chandra S, Pavlick AC. (2012) Targeted therapies for metastatic melanoma. *Dermatol Clin*. 2012 Jul;30(3):517-24; Curti BD, Urba WJ (2012) Integrating new therapies in the treatment of advanced melanoma. *Curr Treat Options Oncol*. 2012 Sep;13(3):327-39.

90 Pajares B, Torres E, Trigo JM, Sáez MI, Ribelles N, Jiménez B, Alba E (2012) Tyrosine kinase inhibitors and drug interactions: a review with practical recommendations. *Clin Transl Oncol*. 2012 Feb;14(2):94-101.

91 Radford IR (2002) Imatinib. Novartis. *Curr Opin Investig Drugs*. 2002 Mar;3(3):492-9.

92 Arteaga CL, Johnson DH (2001) Tyrosine kinase inhibitors-ZD1839 (Iressa). *Curr Opin Oncol*. 2001 Nov;13(6):491-8.

93 Kim TE, Murren JR. (2002) Erlotinib OSI/Roche/Genentech. *Curr Opin Investig Drugs*. 2002 Sep;3(9):1385-95.

94 Kim TE, Murren JR (2003) Lapatinib ditosylate GlaxoSmithKline. *IDrugs*. 2003 Sep;6(9):886-93.

95 Keller G, Schafhausen P, Brümmendorf TH. (2010) Bosutinib. Recent Results *Cancer Res*. 2010;184:119-27.

96 Wissner A, Mansour TS (2008) The development of HKI-272 and related compounds for the treatment of cancer. *Arch Pharm (Weinheim)*. 2008 Aug;341(8):465-77.

97 Drevs J. (2003) PTK/ZK (Novartis). *IDrugs*. 2003 Aug;6(8):787-94.

98 Kumar L (2007) Haematopoietic stem cell transplantation: current status. *Natl Med J India*. 2007 May-Jun;20(3):128-37.

99 Van Zant G, Liang Y (2012) Concise review: hematopoietic stem cell aging, life span, and transplantation. *Stem Cells Transl Med*. 2012 Sep;1(9):651-7.

100 Coleman RE (2012) Adjuvant bone-targeted therapy to prevent metastasis: lessons from the AZURE study. *Curr Opin Support Palliat Care*. 2012 Sep;6(3):322-9.

101 Aapro M, Österborg A, Gascón P, Ludwig H, Beguin Y (2012) Prevalence and management of cancer-related anaemia, iron deficiency and the specific role of i.v. iron. *Ann Oncol*. 2012 Aug;23(8):1954-62.

102 Tonia T, Mettler A, Robert N, Schwarzer G, Seidenfeld J, Weingart O, Hyde C, Engert A, Bohlius J (2012) Erythropoietin or darbepoetin for patients with cancer. *Cochrane Database Syst Rev*. 2012 Dec 12;12:CD003407.

103 Kuehl WM, Bergsagel PL. (2012) Molecular pathogenesis of multiple myeloma and its premalignant precursor. *J Clin Invest*. 2012 Oct 1;122(10):3456-63.

104 Mullen E, Mendez N (2008) Hyperviscosity syndrome in patients with multiple myeloma. *Oncol Nurs Forum*. 2008 May;35(3):350-2.

105 Majhail NS, Lichtin AE (2004) Acute leukemia with a very high leukocyte count: confronting a medical emergency. *Cleve Clin J Med*. 2004 Aug;71(8):633-7.

106 Bisht M, Bist SS, Dhasmana DC (2010) Biological response modifiers: current use and future prospects in cancer therapy. *Indian J Cancer*. 2010 Oct-Dec;47(4):443-51.

107 http://www.macmillan.org.uk/Cancerinformation/Cancertreatment/Treatment types/Supportivetherapies/Steroids.aspx

108 Rosol TJ, Yarrington JT, Latendresse J, Capen CC (2001) Adrenal gland: structure, function, and mechanisms of toxicity. *Toxicol Pathol*. 2001 Jan-Feb;29(1):41-8.

109 Haque SU, Morton D, Welch H. (2012) Biologics against cancer-specific receptors – challenges to personalised medicine from early trial results. *Curr Opin Pharmacol*. 2012 Aug;12(4):392-7; Hoelder S, Clarke PA, Workman P. (2012) Discovery of small molecule cancer drugs: successes, challenges and opportunities. *Mol Oncol*. 2012 Apr;6(2):155-76; Ong FS, Das K, Wang J, Vakil H, Kuo JZ, Blackwell WL, Lim SW, Goodarzi MO, Bernstein KE, Rotter JI, Grody WW. (2012) Personalized medicine and pharmacogenetic biomarkers: progress in molecular oncology testing. *Expert Rev Mol Diagn*. 2012 Jul;12(6):593-602.

110 Podolska K, Stachurska A, Hajdukiewicz K, Małecki M. (2012) Gene therapy prospects--intranasal delivery of therapeutic genes. *Adv Clin Exp Med*. 2012 Jul-Aug;21(4):525-34; Wheeler HE, Maitland ML, Dolan ME, Cox NJ, Ratain MJ. (2013) Cancer pharmacogenomics: strategies and challenges. *Nat Rev Genet*. 2013 Jan;14(1):23-34; Epigenetic therapy: use of agents targeting deacetylation and methylation in cancer management. *OncoTargets and Therapy* 2013:6 223–232.

111 Bollag G, Tsai J, Zhang J, Zhang C, Ibrahim P, Nolop K, Hirth P. (2012) Vemurafenib: the first drug approved for BRAF-mutant cancer. *Nat Rev Drug Discov.* 2012 Nov;11(11):873-86.

112 Dawson MA, Kouzarides T. (2012) Cancer epigenetics: from mechanism to therapy. *Cell.* 2012 Jul 6;150(1):12-27; Popovic R, Licht JD. (2012) Emerging epigenetic targets and therapies in cancer medicine. *Cancer Discov.* 2012 May;2(5):405-13.

113 Zamarin D, Palese P. (2012) Oncolytic Newcastle disease virus for cancer therapy: old challenges and new directions. *Future Microbiol.* 2012 Mar;7(3):347-67; Hoffman RM. (2012) The preclinical discovery of bacterial therapy for the treatment of metastatic cancer with unique advantages. *Expert Opin Drug Discov.* 2012 Jan;7(1):73-83.

114 Amedei A, D'Elios MM. (2012) New therapeutic approaches by using microorganism-derived compounds. *Curr Med Chem.* 2012;19(22):3822-40.

115 Schellmann N, Deckert PM, Bachran D, Fuchs H, Bachran C. (2010) Targeted enzyme prodrug therapies. *Mini Rev Med Chem.* 2010 Sep;10(10):887-904.

116 Alemany R. (2012) Design of improved oncolytic adenoviruses. *Adv Cancer Res.* 2012;115:93-114.

117 Kaneda Y. (2012) Virosome: a novel vector to enable multi-modal strategies for cancer therapy. *Adv Drug Deliv Rev.* 2012 Jun 1;64(8):730-8.

118 Alemany R. (2012) Design of improved oncolytic adenoviruses. *Adv Cancer Res.* 2012;115:93-114.

119 Anand S, Ortel BJ, Pereira SP, Hasan T, Maytin EV. (2012) Biomodulatory approaches to photodynamic therapy for solid tumors. *Cancer Lett.* 2012 Dec 29;326(1):8-16.

120 Patel P, Bryan RT, Wallace DM. (2011) Emerging endoscopic and photodynamic techniques for bladder cancer detection and surveillance. *ScientificWorldJournal.* 2011;11:2550-8.

121 Bhuvaneswari R, Gan YY, Soo KC, Olivo M. (2009) The effect of photodynamic therapy on tumor angiogenesis. *Cell Mol Life Sci.* 2009 Jul;66(14):2275-83.

122 http://www.cancer.gov/cancertopics/factsheet/Therapy/photodynamic

123 Glazer ES, Curley SA. (2011) Non-invasive radiofrequency ablation of malignancies mediated by quantum dots, gold nanoparticles and carbon nanotubes. *Ther Deliv.* 2011 Oct;2(10):1325-30.

124 Abtin FG, Eradat J, Gutierrez AJ, Lee C, Fishbein MC, Suh RD. (2012) Radiofrequency ablation of lung tumors: imaging features of the postablation zone. Radiographics. 2012 Jul-Aug;32(4):947-69.

125 Lencioni R, Crocetti L. (2013) Image-guided ablation for hepatocellular carcinoma. *Recent Results Cancer Res.* 2013;190:181-94.

126 Pai M, Spalding D, Jiao L, Habib N (2012) Use of bipolar radiofrequency in parenchymal transection of the liver, pancreas and kidney. *Dig Surg.* 2012;29(1):43-7.

127 Rosenthal D, Callstrom MR (2012).Critical review and state of the art in interventional oncology: benign and metastatic disease involving bone. *Radiology.* 2012 Mar;262(3):765-80.

128 Volkmer D, Sichlau M, Rapp TB. (2009) The use of radiofrequency ablation in the treatment of musculoskeletal tumors. *J Am Acad Orthop Surg.* 2009 Dec;17(12):737-43.

129 Ahmed M, Moussa M, Goldberg SN. (2012) Synergy in cancer treatment between liposomal chemotherapeutics and thermal ablation. *Chem Phys Lipids.* 2012 May;165(4):424-37.

130 Tang L, Yao C, Sun C. (2009) Apoptosis induction with electric pulses – a new approach to cancer therapy with drug free. *Biochem Biophys Res Commun.* 2009 Dec 25;390(4):1098-101.

131 Chen X, Chen X, Schoenbach KH, Zheng S, Swanson RJ. (2011) Comparative study of long- and short-pulsed electric fields for treating melanoma in an in vivo mouse model. *In Vivo.* 2011 Jan-Feb;25(1):23-7.

132 http://sbirsource.com/sbir/awards/93138-endopulse-system-for-endoscopic-ultrasound-guided-therapy-of-pancreatic-carcinoma

133 Hoff D, Sheikh L, Bhattacharya S, Nayar S, Webster TJ. (2013) Comparison study of ferrofluid and powder iron oxide nanoparticle permeability across the blood-brain barrier. *Int J Nanomedicine.* 2013;8:703-10.

134 Liu HL, Hua MY, Yang HW, Huang CY, Chu PC, Wu JS, Tseng IC, Wang JJ, Yen TC, Chen PY, Wei KC. (2010) Magnetic resonance monitoring of focused ultrasound/magnetic nanoparticle targeting delivery of therapeutic agents to the brain. *Proc Natl Acad Sci U S A.* 2010 Aug 24;107(34):15205-10.

135 Singh S, Sharma A, Robertson GP. (2012) Realizing the clinical potential of cancer nanotechnology by minimizing toxicologic and targeted delivery concerns. *Cancer Res.* 2012 Nov 15;72(22):5663-8.

136 Djamgoz, M.B.A. (2011) Bioelectricity of Cancer, in *The Physiology of Bioelectricity in Development, Tissue Regeneration and Cancer.* Ed., Pullar C.E., *CRC Press, UK.* Pp 269-294; Onkal, R., Djamgoz, M.B.A. (2009) Molecular pharmacology of voltage-gated sodium channel expression in metastatic disease: Clinical potential of neonatal Nav1.5 in breast cancer. *European Journal of Pharmacology,* 25 December 2009, 206–219; Djamgoz MB and Onkal R (2013) Persistent current blockers of voltage-gated sodium channels: a clinical opportunity for controlling metastatic disease. *Recent Pat Anticancer Drug Discov,* 8: 66-84; Brackenbury WJ, Djamgoz MB, Isom LL. (2008) An emerging role for voltage-gated Na+ channels in cellular migration: regulation of central nervous system development and potentiation of invasive cancers. *Neuroscientist.* 2008 Dec;14(6):571-83.

137 Onkal, R., Djamgoz, M.B.A. (2009) Molecular pharmacology of voltage-gated sodium channel expression in metastatic disease: Clinical potential of neonatal Nav1.5 in breast cancer. *European Journal of Pharmacology,* 25 December 2009, 206–219.

138 Djamgoz MB and Onkal R (2013) Persistent current blockers of voltage-gated sodium channels: a clinical opportunity for controlling metastatic disease. *Recent Pat Anticancer Drug Discov,* 8: 66-84; Yang M, Kozminski DJ, Wold LA, Modak R, Calhoun JD, Isom LL, Brackenbury WJ. (2012) Therapeutic potential for phenytoin: targeting Na(v)1.5 sodium channels to reduce migration and invasion in metastatic breast cancer. *Breast Cancer Res Treat.* 2012 Jul;134(2):603-15.

139 Thun MJ, Jacobs EJ, Patrono C. (2012) The role of aspirin in cancer prevention. *Nat Rev Clin Oncol.* 2012 Apr 3;9(5):259-67; Dovizio M, Bruno A, Tacconelli S, Patrignani P. (2013) Mode of action of aspirin as a chemopreventive agent. *Recent Results Cancer Res.* 2013;191:39-65.

140 Djamgoz MB and Onkal R (2013) Persistent current blockers of voltage-gated sodium channels: a clinical opportunity for controlling metastatic disease. *Recent Pat Anticancer Drug Discov,* 8: 66-84.

Step 4 Know Which Complementary Therapies Can Help

1   Tierra, Michael (1998) *The Way of Chinese Herbs.* Simon & Schuster.

2   Smith, M.E., Bauer-Wu, S. (2012) Traditional Chinese Medicine for cancer-related symptoms. *Seminars in Oncology Nursing*, 28 (1), 64-74; Lee SK, Dawson J, Lee JA, Osman G, Levitin M, Guzel RM & Djamgoz MBA. Cancer pain: Integrative management approaches and their wider implications. MS submitted; Paley CA, Johnson MI, Tashani OA, Bagnall AM (2011). Acupuncture for cancer pain in adults. *Cochrane Database of Systematic Reviews*, Issue 1. Art. No.: CD007753. DOI: 10.1002/14651858.CD007753.pub2; Shukla S, Torossian A, Duann JR, Leung A. (2011) The analgesic effect of electroacupuncture on acute thermal pain perception – a central neural correlate study with fMRI. *Mol Pain*, 7:45; Sima L & Yin C (2009). Efficacy of electroacupuncture for bone metastatic cancer patients with neuropathic pain: A randomized controlled trial. *J Clin Oncol*, 27:15(suppl; abstr 9534).

3   Lee SK, Dawson J, Lee JA, Osman G, Levitin M, Guzel RM & Djamgoz MBA. Cancer pain: Integrative management approaches and their wider implications. MS submitted.

4   Sima L & Yin C (2009). Efficacy of electroacupuncture for bone metastatic cancer patients with neuropathic pain: A randomized controlled trial. *J Clin Oncol*, 27:15(suppl; abstr 9534).

5   Paley CA, Johnson MI, Tashani OA, Bagnall AM (2011). Acupuncture for cancer pain in adults. *Cochrane Database of Systematic Reviews*, Issue 1. Art. No.: CD007753. DOI: 10.1002/14651858.CD007753.pub2.

6   Shukla S, Torossian A, Duann JR, Leung A. (2011) The analgesic effect of electroacupuncture on acute thermal pain perception – a central neural correlate study with fMRI. *Mol Pain*, 7:45.

7   http://www.dailymail.co.uk/health/article-1254746/Chinese-medicine-caused-kidney-failure-cancer-So-safe-popular-cures.html

8   Coghlan ML et al. (2012) Deep Sequencing of Plant and Animal DNA Contained Within Traditional Chinese Medicines Reveals Legality Issues and Health Safety Concerns. *PLOS Genetics*; Toxic Poisoning Alert for Online Chinese Medicines. MHRA. 2013; Public Health Risk with Herbal Medicines: an Overview. MHRA. 2008; see regular MHRA safety alerts.

9   Pakade, Y.B., Kumari, A., Singh, S., Sharma, R., Tewary, D.K. (2011) Metals in Herbal Drugs from Himalayan Region. *Bulletin of Environmental Contamination and Toxicology,* 86 (1), 133-136; Gunturu, K.S., Nagarajan, P., McPhedran, P., Goodman, T.R., Hodsdon, M.E., Strout, M.P. (2011) Ayurvedic herbal medicine and lead poisoning. *Journal of Hematology & Oncology,* 4,51; Nnorom, I.C. Osibanjo, O., Eleke, C. (2006). Evaluation of human exposure to lead and cadmium from some local Nigerian medicinal preparations. *Journal of Applied Sciences*, 6 (14). 2907-2911.

10 Chen, C-H., Dickman, K.G., Moriya, M., Zavadil, J., Sidorenko, V.S., Edwards, K.L. et al. (2012) Aristolochic acid-associated urothelial cancer in Taiwan. *Proceedings of the National Academy of Sciences of the United States of America, 109 (21) 8241-8246.*

11 Plant, Jane, 2007. *Your Life in Your Hands*. Fourth edition. Virgin Books; Plant, Jane (2007) *Understand, prevent and overcome prostate cancer*. Revised edition. Virgin Books; Goldacre, Ben (2012) *Bad Pharma: How drug companies mislead doctors and harm patients*. Fourth Estate; Mayor, Susan (2002) Researchers claim clinical trials are reported with misleading statistics. *BMJ*, 324, 1353; *JAMA* (2003) 389, 454-465, quoted by Hopkins Tanne, Janice (2003) Industry is deeply involved in funding US research. *BMJ*, 326, 179; Tonks, Alison (2002) Authors of guidelines have strong links with drugs industry. *BMJ*, 324, 383.

12 Crespo-Ortiz MP & Wei MQ (2012). Antitumor activity of artemisinin and its derivatives: from a well-known antimalarial agent to a potential anticancer drug. *J Biomed Biotechnol*, 2012:247597. doi: 10.1155/2012/247597.

13 Laszczyk MN (2009). Pentacyclic triterpenes of the lupane, oleanane and ursane group as tools in cancer therapy. *Planta Med*, 75:1549-60.

14 Bar-Sela G, Wollner M, Hammer L, Agbarya A, Dudnik E & Haim N (2012). Mistletoe as complementary treatment in patients with advanced non-small-cell lung cancer treated with carboplatin-based combinations: A randomised phase II study. *Eur J Cancer*, doi: 10.1016/j.ejca.2012.11.007. [Epub ahead of print.]

15 Jin X, Ruiz Beguerie J, Sze DM & Chan GC (2012). *Ganoderma lucidum* (Reishi mushroom) for cancer treatment. *Cochrane Database Syst Rev*, Jun 13;6:CD007731.

16 Frenkel M, Mishra BM, Sen S, Yang P, Pawlus A, Vence L, Leblanc A, Cohen L, Banerji P & Banerji P (2010). Cytotoxic effects of ultra-diluted remedies on breast cancer cells. *Int J Oncol*, 36:395-403.

17 Servan Schreiber, David (2011) *Healing Without Freud or Prozac: Natural approaches to curing stress, anxiety and depression*. Rodale.

18 http://www.cancerresearchuk.org/cancer-help/about-cancer/treatment/complementary-alternative/therapies/hypnotherapy#evidence

19 Elkins, G., Marcus, J., Stearns, V., Rajab, M.H. (2007) Pilot evaluation of hypnosis for the treatment of hot flashes in breast cancer survivors. *Psycho-Oncology*, 16 (5), 487-492; www.cancerresearchuk.org

20 Tome-Pires, C., Miro, J. (2012) Hypnosis for the management of chronic and cancer procedure- related pain in children. *International Journal of Clinical and Experimental Hypnosis*, 60 (4), 432-457.

21 Zeidan F, Martucci KT, Kraft RA, Gordon NS, McHaffie JG, Coghill RC (2011). Brain mechanisms supporting the modulation of pain by mindfulness meditation. *J Neurosci* 31:5540-5548.

22 Grant JA, Courtemanche J, Duerden EG, Duncan GH & Rainville P (2010). Cortical thickness and pain sensitivity in Zen meditators. *Emotion*, 10:43–53.

23 Zeidan F, Martucci KT, Kraft RA, Gordon NS, McHaffie JG, Coghill RC (2011). Brain mechanisms supporting the modulation of pain by mindfulness meditation. *J Neurosci* 31:5540-5548.

24 http://www.cancerresearchuk.org/cancer-help/about-cancer/treatment/complementary-alternative/therapies/visualisation

25 http://www.cancerresearchuk.org/cancer-help/about-cancer/treatment/complementary-alternative/therapies/visualisation

26 Cancer Research UK trial no CRUK/03/025.

27 Yeom et al., 2009

28 Vollbracht et al., 2011

29 Monti et al., 2012

30 Yan Ma et al(2014). High-Dose Parenteral Ascorbate Enhanced Chemosensitivity of Ovarian Cancer and Reduced Toxicity of Chemotherapy. Sci Transl Med 6, 222ra18 (2014)

31 http://www.cancer.org/treatment/treatmentsandsideeffects/complementaryandalternativemedicine/herbsvitaminsandminerals/essiac-tea

32 Schauss, A.G., (1991) Nephrotoxicity and neurotoxicity in humans from organogermanium compounds and germanium dioxide. *Biological Trace Element Research*, 29 (3), 267-280; http://curezone.com/diseases/cancer/germanium.asp; http://www.cancer.org/treatment/treatmentsandsideeffects/complementaryandalternativemedicine/herbsvitaminsandminerals/germanium

33 http://www.gerson.org

34 http://www.cancer.org/Treatment/TreatmentsandSideEffects/Complementary andAlternativeMedicine/DietandNutrition/gerson-therapy)

35 Chabot, J.A., Tsai, W-Y., Fine, R.L. (2010) Pancreatic proteolytic enzyme therapy compared with gemcitabine-based chemotherapy for the treatment of pancreatic cancer. *Journal of Clinical Oncology* 28 (12), 2058-2063.

36 Larrick, G.P., (1956). Public Warning Against Hoxsey cancer treatment: Food and Drug Administration Washington 25, D.C. *Canadian Medical Association Journal,* 74 (9), 740; Larrick, G.P., (1957). Statement on Hoxsey cancer treatment. *Journal of the National Medical Association.* 49 (2) 123; Hoxsey Herbal Treatment, American Cancer Society; Herbal / Plant Therapies: Hoxsey, from the Department of Complementary and Integrative Medicine of M. D. Anderson Cancer Center; Hoxsey Herbal Therapy, from the Memorial Sloan-Kettering Cancer Center; This Week in FDA History, U.S. Food and Drug Administration.

37 Matsumoto et al., (2009) Simultaneous imaging of tumor oxygenation and microvascular permeability using Overhauser enhanced MRI. *Proc. Natl. Acad. Sci. USA*; 106(42): 17,898-17,903; Bourke et al., (2007) Correlation of radiation response with tumor oxygenation in the Dunning prostate R3327-AT1 tumor. *Int. J. Radiat. Oncol. Biol. Phys.*67(4): 1179-1186; Kodibagkar et al., (2008) Proton imaging of siloxanes to map tissue oxygenation levels (PISTOL): a tool for quantitative tissue oximetry. *NMR Biomed.* 21(8): 899–907; Avni R, Cohen B and Neeman M (2011) Hypoxic stress and cancer: imaging the axis of evil in tumor metastasis. *NMR Biomed*; Golman *et al.,* (2006) Metabolic imaging by hyperpolarized 13C magnetic resonance imaging for in vivo tumor diagnosis. *Cancer Res.* 66(22): 10,855-10,860; Catana *et al.,* (2008) Simultaneous in vivo positron emission tomography and magnetic resonance imaging. *Proc. Natl. Acad. Sci. USA*,105(10): 3705-3710; Golman et al., (2006) Metabolic imaging by hyperpolarized 13C magnetic resonance imaging for in vivo tumor diagnosis. *Cancer Res.* 66(22): 10,855-10,860; Gallagher et al., (2008) Magnetic resonance imaging of pH in vivo using hyperpolarized 13C labelled bicarbonate. *Nature.* 453(7197): 940-943; Brown J.M. & Wilson W.R 2004 *Nature Reviews Cancer* 4, 437-447.

38 http://www.nhs.uk/Conditions/photodynamic-therapy-NGPDT-sonodynamic-therapy/Pages/Introduction.aspx

39 de Mejia EG, Dia VP (2010) The role of nutraceutical proteins and peptides in apoptosis, angiogenesis, and metastasis of cancer cells. *Cancer and Metastasis Reviews*, 29, 511-528.

Step 5 Eat to Beat Cancer

1 Doll, R., Peto, R. (1981) The causes of cancer: quantitative estimates of avoidable risks of cancer in the United States today. *Journal of the National Cancer Institute*, 66 (6), 1191-1308.

2 Block, G., Patterson, B., Subar, A. (1992) Fruit, vegetables, and cancer prevention: a review of the epidemiological evidence. *Nutrition and Cancer*, 18 (1), 1-29.

3 Campbell, C. T., Campbell, T. M. (2006) *The China Study: the most comprehensive study of nutrition ever conducted and the starting implications for diet, weight loss and long-term health.* Dallas, Texas. BenBella Books.

4 Chan, J. M., Giovannucci, E. L. (2001) Dairy products, calcium, and vitamin D and risk of prostate cancer. *Epidemiological Reviews*, 23 (1), 87-92; Sinha, R., Anderson, D. E., McDonald, S. S., Greenwald, P. (2003) Cancer risk and diet in India. *Journal of Postgraduate Medicine*, 49, 222-228; Potter, J. D., McMichael,

A. J. (1986) Diet and cancer of the colon and rectum: a case-control study. *Journal of the National Cancer Institute*, 76 (4), 557-569.

5   Carroll, K.K. (1975) Experimental evidence of dietary factors and hormone-dependent factors. *Cancer Research*, 35, 3374-3383.

6   Ferrucci, L., Sinha, R., Huang, W et al. (2012) Meat consumption and the risk of incident distal colon rectal adenoma. *British journal of Cancer,* 106: 3: 608-616.

7   Ibiebele, T., Hughes, M., Whiteman, D., Webb, P. (2011) Dietary patterns and risk of Oesophageal cancers: a population-based case-control study. *Br J Nutr.* Sep 7:1-10; Bravi et al, (2011) Dietary patterns and risk of oesophageal cancer. *Annals of oncology*, 06/10/2011.

8   Wang, C. et al (2011) Meat intake and risk of bladder cancer: a meta-analysis. *Medical Oncology.* 19/06/2011.

9   Sinha, R. Park, Y., Graubard, M., Leitzmann, M., Hollenbeck, A., Schatzkin, A., Cross, A. (2009) Meat and Meat related compounds and risk of prostate cancer in a large prospective cohort study in the United states. *American Journal of epidemiology.* 170, 9 1165-1177; Richman, E., Kenfield, S., Stampfer, M., Giovannucci, E., Chan, J. (2011) *Cancer Prev Res* (Phila). Dec;4(12):2110-21.

10 Jakszyn, P., Agudo, A. et al, Gonzalez, C. (2012) Dietary intake of heme iron and risk of gastric cancer in the European prospective investigation into cancer and nutrition study. *Int J Cancer.* Jun 1;130 (11):2654-63.

11 Blank, M., Wentzensen, N., Murphy, M., Hollenbeck, A., Park, Y. (2012) Dietary fat intake and risk of ovarian cancer in the NIH-AARP Diet and Health Study. *British Journal of cancer*:106:3:596-602.

12 Stoneham, L. (2012) Cancer loves red meat. Published Jan 14, 2012; Fiore, K. (2012) Bacon, Sausage Linked to Pancreatic Cancer. MedPage today. Published Jan 13, 2012; http;//www.naturalnews.com/032890_red_meat_food_additives.html; http://www.naturalnews.com/030050_dentist_cancer.html

13 Ibiebele, T., Hughes, M., Whiteman, D., Webb, P. (2011) Dietary patterns and risk of Oesophageal cancers: a population-based case-control study. *Br J Nutr.* Sep 7:1-10.

14 Piyathilake, C.J., Badiga, S., Kabagambe, E.K., Azuero, A., Alvarez, R.D., Johanning, G.L., Partridge, E.E. (2012) Dietary Pattern Associated with LINE-1 Methylation Alters the Risk of Developing Cervical Intraepithelial Neoplasia. *Cancer Prevention Research*, 5 (3), 385-392.

15 Levine, M. E., Suarez, J.A., Brandhorst, S., Balasubramanian, P., Cheng, C., Madia, F., Fontana, L., Mirisola, M.G., Guevara-Aguirre, J., Wan, J., Passarino, G., Kennedy, B.K., Wei, M., Cohen, P., Crimmins, E.M., Longo, V.D. (2014) Low Protein Intake Is Associated with a Major Reduction in IGF-1, Cancer, and Overall Mortality in the 65 and Younger but Not Older Population. *Cell Metabolism*, Volume 19, Issue 3, 407-417, 4 March 2014.

16 Campbell, C. T., Campbell, T. M. (2006) *The China Study: the most comprehensive study of nutrition ever conducted and the starting implications for diet, weight loss and long-term health.* Dallas, Texas. BenBella Books.

17 NDNS (2002) The national diet & nutrition survey: adults aged 19 to 64 years. Types and quantities of food consumed. Volume 1.

18 Humphrys, J. (2002) *The great food gamble: What we are doing to our food and how it affects our health.* United Kingdom. Hodder & Stoughton.

19 Schlosser, E. (2002) *Fast Food Nation: the dark side of the all-American meal.* London, England. Penguin Books.

20 Moschen, Alexander R., Wieser ,Verena, Tilg, Herbert (2012) Dietary Factors: Major Regulators of the Gut's Microbiota. *Gut Liver*, 6(4) 411-416.

21 Ornish, D.M., Magbanua, M. J. M., Weidner, G., Weinberg, V., Kemp, C., Green, C., Mattie, M., Marlin, R., Simko, J., Shinohara, K., Haqq, C. M., Carroll, P. R. (2008) Changes in prostate gene expression in men undergoing an intensive nutrition and lifestyle intervention. *Proceedings of the National Academy of Sciences*, 105 (24), 8369-8374.

22 Plant, J., Tidey, G. (2004) *The Plant Programme – recipes for fighting breast and prostate cancer*. London, UK. Virgin Books.

23 Herbert, J. et al (2012) A diet, physical activity and stress reduction intervention in men with rising prostate-specific antigen after treatment for prostate cancer. *Cancer epidemiology* 28/3/2012.

24 Fidler, I. J. (1995) Modulation of the organ microenvironment for treatment of cancer metastasis. *Journal of the National Cancer Institute*, 87 (21), 1588-1592; Fidler, I. J. (2003) The pathogenesis of cancer metastasis: the 'seed and soil' hypothesis revisited. *Nature Reviews – Cancer*, 3, 1-6; Paget, S. (1889) The distribution of secondary growths in cancer of the breast. *Lancet*, 1, 571-573.

25 Organ, C., Nunn, C. L., Machanda, Z., Wrangham, R. W. (2011) Phylogenetic rate shifts in feeding time during the evolution of *Homo*. *Proceedings of the National Academy of Sciences*, 108 (35), 14555-14559.

26 Plant, Jane, Tidey, Gill (2010) *Eating for Better Health*. Virgin Books.

27 Lin, J. et al (2012) Intake of red meat and heterocyclic amines, metabolic pathway genes, and bladder cancer risk. *International Journal of Cancer* 7/3/2012.

28 Daniel, C., Schwartz, K., Colt, J., Dong, L., Ruterbusch, J., Purdue, M., Cross, A., Rothman, N., Davis, F., Wacholder, S., Graubard, B., Chow, W., Sinha, R. (2011) Meat-cooking mutagens and risk of renal cell carcinoma. *British journal of cancer* 105,1096-1104.

29 Fenske, R. R. (2005) State-of-the-art measurement of agricultural pesticide exposures. *Scandinavian Journal of Work, Environment and Health*, 31, 67-73; Lu, C., Toepel, K., Irish, R., Fenske, R. A., Barr, D. B., Bravo, R. (2006) Organic diets significantly lower children's dietary exposure to organophosphorus pesticides. *Environmental Health Perspectives*, 114 (2), 260-263.

30 Jong, F. M. W., Snoo, G. R. (2001) Pesticide residues in human food and wildlife in the Netherlands. *Mededelingen Faculteit Landbouwkundige en Toegepaste Biologische Wetenschappen Universiteit Gent*, 66 (2B), 815-822; Newsome, W. H., Doucet, J., Davies, D., Sun, W. F. (2000) Pesticide residues in the Canadian market basket survey – 1992-1996. *Food additives and contaminants*, 17 (10), 847-854; Poulsen, M. E., Andersen, J. H. (2003) Results from the monitoring of pesticide residues in fruit and vegetables on the Danish market, 2000-01. *Food Additives and Contaminants*, 20 (8), 742-757.

31 Stepan, R. R. (2005) Baby food production chain: pesticide residues in fresh apples and products. *Food Additives and Contaminants*, 22 (12), 1231-1242.

32 Jong FMW, et al. (2001) Pesticide residues in human food and wildlife in the Netherlands. *Mededelingen Faculteit Landbouwkundige en Toegepaste Biologische Wetenschappen Universiteit Gent*, 66 (2B), 815-822; Herrera A, et al. (1996) Estimates of mean daily intakes of persistent organochlorine pesticides from Spanish fatty foodstuffs. *Bulletin of Environmental Contamination and Toxicology*, 56 (2), 173-177.

33 Charlier, C. J., Plomteux, G. J. (2002) Determination of organochlorine pesticide residues in the blood of healthy individuals. *Clinical Chemisrty and*

Laboratory Medicine, 40 (4), 361-364; Dewailly, E., Mulvad, G., Pedersen, H. S., Ayotte, P. S., Demers, A., Weber, J-P., Hansen, J. C. (1999) Concentration of organochlorines in human brain, liver, and adipose tissue autopsy samples from Greenland. *Environmental Health Perspectives*, 107 (10), 823-828; Nakagawa, R., Hirakawa, H., Iida, T., Matsueda, T., Nagayama, J. (1999) Maternal body burden of organochlorine pesticides and dioxins. *The Journal of AOAC International*, 82 (3), 716-724; Olea, N., Olea-Serrano, F., Lardelli-Claret, P., Rivas, A., Barba-Navarro, A. (1999) Inadvertent exposure to xenoestrogens in children. *Toxicology and Industrial Health*, 15 (1–2), 151-158.

34 Bro-Rasmussen, F. (1996) Contamination by persistent chemicals in food chain and human health. *Science of the Total Environment*, 188, S45-S60; Darnerud, P. O., Atuma, S., Aune, M., Bjerselius, R., Glynn, A., Petersson Grawé, K., Becker, W. (2006) Dietry intake estimations of organohalogen contaminants (dioxins, PCB, PBDE and chlorinated pesticides, e. g. DDT) based on Swedish market based data. *Food and Chemical Toxicology*, 44 (9), 1597-1606.

35 McKinlay, R., Dassyne, J., Djamgoz, M. B. A., Plant, J., Voulvoulis, N. (2012) Agricultural pesticides and chemical fertilisers. In: Plant, J. A., Voulvoulis, N. & Ragnarsdottir, K. V. (eds.) *Pollutants, human health and the environment: a risk based approach*. Wiley. 181-206.

36 Birnbaum, L. S., Fenton, S. E. (2003) Cancer and development exposure to endocrine disruptors. *Environmental Health Perspectives*, 111 (4), 389-394.

37 Diamanti-Kandarakis, E., Bourguignon, J-P., Giudice, L. C., Hauser, R., Prins, G. S., Soto, A. M., Zoeller, R. T., Gore, A. C. (2009) Endocrine-disrupting chemicals: an endocrine society scientific statement. *Endocrine Reviews*, 30 (4), 293-342.

38 Beaton C. (Ed.) (2006) *The Farm Management Handbook 2006/7*. Edinburgh: Scottish Agricultural College.

39 Givens, M.L., Lu, C., Bartell, S.M., Pearson, M.A. (2006) Estimating dietary consumption patterns among children: a comparison between cross-sectional and longitudinal study designs. *Environmental Research*, 99 (3), 1065-1079.

40 Pesticide Action Network (2006) *Pesticides in your food*. [Online.] Available from: http://www.pan-uk.org/archive/Projects/Food/index.htm [Accessed 1st May 2012].

41 McKinlay, R., Dassyne, J., Djamgoz, M.B.A., Plant, J., Voulvoulis, N. (2012) Agricultural pesticides and chemical fertilisers. In: Plant, J. A., Voulvoulis, N. & Ragnarsdottir, K.V. (eds.) *Pollutants, human health and the environment: a risk based approach*. Wiley. 181-206.

42 Campbell, C.T., Junshi, C. (1994) Diet and chronic degenerative disease perspectives from China. *American Journal of Clinical Nutrition*, 59, 1153S-1161S.

43 Atkins, R.C. (1972) *Dr. Atkins' Diet Revolution*. Bantam Books; Pritikin, R. (1973) *The Pritikin Principle: The Calorie Density Solution*.

44 Hamilton, M., Greenway, F. (2004) Evaluating commercial weight loss programmes: an evolution in outcomes research. *Obesity Reviews*, 5 (4), 217-232.

45 Atkins, R.C. (1972) *Dr. Atkins' Diet Revolution*. Bantam Books.

46 Dunaif, G.E., Campbell, T.C. (1987) Relative contribution of dietary protein level and aflatoxin B1 dose in generation of presumptive preneoplastic foci in rat liver. *Journal of the National Cancer Institute*, 78, 365-369; Youngman, L. D., Campbell, T.C. (1992) Inhibition of aflatoxin B1-induced gamma-glutamyl transpeptidase positive (GGT) hepatic preneoplastic foci and tumors by low

protein diets: evidence that altered GGT foci indicate neoplastic potential. *Carcinogenesis*, 13, 1607-1613.

47 Campbell, C.T., Junshi, C. (1994) Diet and chronic degenerative disease perspectives from China. *American Journal of Clinical Nutrition*, 59, 1153S-1161S.

48 http://dx.doi.org/10.1038/nature12968

49 Remer, T., Manz, F. (1994) Potential renal acid load of foods and its influence on urine pH. *Journal of the American Dietetic Association*, 95 (7), 791-797.

50 Campbell, C.T., Campbell, T.M. (2006) *The China Study: the most comprehensive study of nutrition ever conducted and the starting implications for diet, weight loss and long-term health*. Dallas, Texas. BenBella Books; Esselstyn Jr., C. B. (2008) *Prevent and reverse heart disease: The revolutionary, scientifically proven, nutrition-based cure*. USA. Penguin Group; Ganmaa, D., Sato, A. (2005) Possible role of female sex hormones in milk from pregnant cows in the development of breast, ovarian and corpus uteri cancers. *Medical Hypothesis*, 65 (6), 1028-1037; McDougall, J. A. (1991) *The McDougall programme: Twelve days to dynamic health*. Plume Books. USA. Penguin Group.

51 Martin, O.V., Evans, R.M (2012) Naturally occurring oestrogens. In: Plant, J. A., Voulvoulis, N. & Ragnarsdottir, K.V. (eds.) *Pollutants, human health and the environment: a risk based approach*. Wiley, 229-254.

52 Campbell, C.T., Campbell, T.M. (2006) *The China Study: the most comprehensive study of nutrition ever conducted and the starting implications for diet, weight loss and long-term health*. Dallas, Texas. BenBella Books; Ganmaa, D., Sato, A. (2005) Possible role of female sex hormones in milk from pregnant cows in the development of breast, ovarian and corpus uteri cancers. *Medical Hypothesis*, 65 (6), 1028-1037.

53 Handa, Y., Fujita, H., Honma, S., Minakami, H., Kishi, R. (2009) Estrogen concentrations in beef and human hormone-dependent cancers. *Annals of Oncology*, 20 (9), 1610-1611.

54 Campbell, C.T., Campbell, T.M. (2006) *The China Study: the most comprehensive study of nutrition ever conducted and the starting implications for diet, weight loss and long-term health*. Dallas, Texas. BenBella Books.

55 Butler, J. (2007) *One in nine. The VVF ask why breast cancer cases are rising and investigates the role of diet*. [Online]. Available from: http://www.fishpond.co.nz/Books/One-Nine-Justine-Butler/9780955765308?cf=3 [Accessed 1st May 2012].

56 Harvard Medical School: Harvard Health Publications (2008) *Healthy Eating Plate*. [Online]. Available from: http://www.hsph.harvard.edu/nutritionsource/what-should-you-eat/pyramid [Accessed 4th April 2012].

57 Campbell, C.T., Campbell, T.M. (2006) *The China Study: the most comprehensive study of nutrition ever conducted and the starting implications for diet, weight loss and long-term health*. Dallas, Texas. BenBella Books.

58 Azzouz, A., Jurado-Sanchez, B., Souhail, B., Ballesteros, E. (2011) Simultaneous dtermination of 20 Pharmacologically active substances in cow's milk, goat's milk and human breast milk by Gas chromatography – Mass spectrometry. *J Agricultural and Food Chemistry*. 59,5125-5132.

59 LeRoith, D., Helman, L. (2004) The new kid on the block(ade) of the IGF-1 receptor. *Cancer Cell*, 5 (3), 201-202; Wolk, A., Bergström, R., Mantzoros, C. S., Lagiou, P., Andersson, S-O., Signorello, L.B., Trichopoulos, D., Adami, H-O. (1998) Insulin-like growth factor 1 and prostate cancer risk: a population-based, case control study. *Journal of the National Cancer Institute*, 90 (12), 911-

915; Wu, Y., Cui, K., Miyoshi, K., Hennighausen, L., Green, J. E., Sester, J., LeRoith, D., Yakar, S. (2003) Reduced circulating insulin-like growth factor I levels delay the onset of chemically and genetically induced mammary tumors. *Cancer Research*, 63 (15), 4383-4388; Yu, H., Rohan, T. (2000) Role of insulin-like growth factor family in cancer development and progression. *Journal of the National Cancer Institute*, 92 (18), 1472-1489.

60 Holly, J. (2004) IGF-1, IGFBP-3, and cancer risk. *The Lancet*, 364 (9431), 325-326.

61 Chan, J.M., Stampfer, M.J., Ma, J., Gann, P., Gaziano, M.J., Pollak, M., Giovannucci, E. (2002) Insulin-like growth factor-I (IGF-1) and IGF binding protein-3 as predictors of advanced-stage prostate cancer. *Journal of the National Cancer Institute*, 94 (14), 1099-1106.

62 Holmes, M.D., Pollak, M.N., Willett, W.C., Hankinson, S.E. (2002) Dietary correlates of plasma insulin-like growth factor I and insulin-like growth factor binding protein 3 concentrations. *Cancer Epidemiology, Biomarkers & Prevention*, 11, 852-861; Kaklamani, V.G., Linos, A., Kaklamani, E., Markaki, I., Koumantaki, Y., Mantzoros, C.S. (1999) Dietary fat and carbohydrates are independently associated with circulating insulin-like growth factor 1 and insulin-like growth factor-binding protein 3 concentrations in healthy adults. *Journal of Clinical Oncology*, 17, 3291-3298; Ma, J., Giovannucci, E., Pollak, M., Chan, J. M., Gaziano, J. M., Willett, W., Stampfer, M. J. (2001) Milk intake, circulating levels of insulin-like growth factor-i, and risk of colorectal cancer in men. *Journal of the National Cancer Institute*, 93, 1330-1336.

63 Allen, N.E., Appleby, P.N., Davey, G.K., Key, T.J. (2000) Hormones and diet: low insulin-like growth factor-I but normal bioavailable androgens in vegan men. *British Journal of Cancer*, 83 (1), 95-97.

64 Allen N.E, Appleby, P.N., Davey, G.K., Kaaks, R., Rinaldi, S., Key, T.J. (2002) The associations of diet with serum insulin-like growth factor I and its main binding proteins in 292 women meat-eaters, vegetarians, and vegans. *Cancer Epidemiology, Biomarkers & Prevention*, 11 (11), 1441-1448.

65 Bradley, A.J., Leach, K.A., Breen, J.E., Green, L.E., Green, M.J. (2007) Survey of the incidence and aetiology of mastitis on dairy farms in England and Wales. *Veterinary Record*, 160, 253-258.

66 Echternkamp, S.E., Vonnahme, K.A., Green, J.A., Ford, S.P. (2006) Increased vascular endothelial growth factor and pregnancy-associated glycoproteins, but not insulin-like growth factor-I, in maternal blood of cows gestating twins foetuses. *Journal of Animal Science*, 84 (8), 2057-2064.

67 Hymowitz, T. (1970) On the domestication of the soybean. *Economic Botany*, 24 (4), 408-421.

68 *The Book of Tofu*, William Sirtleff and Akiko Aoyagi 1975 (Autumn Press Inc).

69 Martin, O.V., Evans, R.M (2012) Naturally occurring oestrogens. In: Plant, J.A., Voulvoulis, N. & Ragnarsdottir, K.V. (eds.) *Pollutants, human health and the environment: a risk based approach*. Wiley, 229-254.

70 Milligan, S.R., Kalita, J.C., Pocock, V., Van De Kauter, V., Stevens, J.F., Deinzer, M.L., Rong, H., De Keukeleire, D. (2000) The endocrine activities of 8-prenylnaringenin and related hop (*Humulus lupulus L.*) flavonoids. *The Journal of Clinical Endocrinology & Metabolism*, 85, 4912-4915.

71 Mersereau, J.E., Levy, N., Staub, R.E., Baggett, S., Zogric, T., Chow, S., Ricke, W.A., Tagliaferri, M., Cohen, I., Bjeldanes, L.F., Leitman, D.C. (2008) Liquiritigenin is a plant-derived highly selective estrogen receptor [beta agonist.] *Molecular and Cellular Endocrinology*, 283, 49-57.

72 Allred K.F., Yackley, K.M., Vanamala, J., Allred, C.D. (2009). Trigonelline is a novel phytoestrogen in coffee beans. *The Journal of Nutrition*, 139 (10), 1833-1836.

73 Martin, O.V., Evans, R.M (2012) Naturally occurring oestrogens. In: Plant, J. A., Voulvoulis, N. & Ragnarsdottir, K.V. (eds.) *Pollutants, human health and the environment: a risk based approach*. Wiley, 229-254.

74 Martin, O.V., Evans, R.M (2012) Naturally occurring oestrogens. In: Plant, J. A., Voulvoulis, N. & Ragnarsdottir, K.V. (eds.) *Pollutants, human health and the environment: a risk based approach*. Wiley, 229-254.

75 Miyanaga, N., Akaza, H., Hinotsu, S., Fujioka, T., Naito, S., Namiki, M.et al, Tsuji, H. (2011) A prostate cancer Chemoprevention study: An investigative Randomized control study using purified Isoflavones in men with rising PSA. Cancer science. DOI: 10.1111/j.1349-7006.2011.02120.x.

76 Mann, D. (2011) Is Soy safe to eat after breast cancer? WEB MD Health News.

77 Ollberding, N., Lim, U., Wilkens, L., Setiawan, V., Shvetsov, Y., Henderson, B., Kolonel, L., Goodman, M. (2012) Legume, Soy, Tofu and Isoflavone intake and endometrial cancer in postmenopausal women in the multi-ethnic cohort study. *J Natl Cancer Inst*. 2012 Jan 4;104(1):67-76. Epub 2011 Dec 12.

78 http://www.vegetarian.org.uk/factsheets/safetyofsoya.html

79 Aune, D., Chan, D., Greenwood, D., Vieira, A., Rosenblatt, D., Vieira, R., Norat, T. (2012) Dietary fiber and breast cancer risk: a systematic review and meta-analysis of prospective studies. *Ann Oncol*. Feb 3 [Epub ahead of print]; Zhang, C., Ho, S., Cheng, S., Chen, Y., Fu, J., Lin, F. (2011) Effect of dietary fiber intake on breast cancer risk according to estrogen and progesterone receptor status. *European Journal of Clinical Nutrition*. 65, 929-936.

80 McCarty, M. (1999) Vegan proteins may reduce cancer risk of cancer, obesity, and cardiovascular disease by promoting increased glucagon activity. *Med Hypotheses*. Dec;53(6):459-85.

81 Plant, Jane, Tidey, Gill (2010) *Eating for Better Health*. Virgin Books.

82 Simopoulos, A.P. (2002) The importance of the ratio of omega-6/omega-3 essential fatty acids. *Biomedicine & Pharmacotherapy*, 56 (8), 365-379.

83 Warburg, O.H. (1966) The prime cause and prevention of cancer: part 1.

84 For further information see also Plant, Jane, Tidey, Gill (2010) *Eating for Better Health* (Virgin Books) and Plant, Jane, 2007 *Your Life in Your Hands*. Fourth edition (Virgin Books).

85 Jihn Yudkin, 1972, *Pure, White and Deadly*. First published in 1972; reissued by Penguin Books in 2013.

86 Lu, J., Zhang, K., Nam, S., Anderson, R.A., Jove, R., Wen, W. (2010) Novel angiogenesis inhibitory activity in cinnamon extract blocks VEGFR2 kinase and downstream signalling. *Carcinogenesis*, 31 (3), 481-488.

87 López-Lázaro, M. (2009) Distribution and biological activities of the flavonoid luteolin. *Mini-Reviews in Medicinal Chemistry*, 9 (1), 31-59; Shimoi, K., Okada, H., Furugori, M., Goda, T., Takase, S., Suzuki, M., Hara, Y., Yamamoto, H., Kinae, N. (1998) Intestinal absorption of luteolin and luteolin 7-0-[beta]-glucoside in rats and humans. *FEBS Letters*, 438 (3), 220-224.

88 Zheng, G-q., Kenney, P.M., Zhang, J., Lam, L.K.T. (1992) Inhibition of benzo[*a*] pyrene-induced tumorigenesis by myristicin, a volatile aroma constituent of parsley leaf oil. *Carcinogenesis*, 13 (10), 1921-1923.

89 Li, W. (2010) Can we eat to starve cancer [Video USA, TED Conferences.]

90 Reinmann C & Birke (eds) Geochemistry of European bottled water Birntrtraegerscience pub. Stuttgart.

91 Klag, M. J., Wang, N.Y., Meoni, L.A., Brancati, F.L., Cooper, L.A., Liany, K.Y., Young, Y.H., Ford, D.E. (2002) Coffee intake and risk of hypertension; the Johns Hopkins precursors study. *Archives of Internal Medicine*, 162 (6), 657-662.

92 Rodriguez, T., Rodriguez, T., Altieri, A., Chatenoud, L., Gallus, S., Bosetti, C., Negri, E., Franceschi, S., Levi, F., Talamini, R., La Vecchia, C. (2004) Risk factors for oral and pharyngeal cancer in young adults. *Oral Oncology*, 42 (2), 207-213; Tavani, A., Bertuzzi, M., Talamini, R., Gallus, S., Parpinel, M., Franceschi, S., Levi, F., La Vecchia, C. (2003) Coffee and tea intake and risk of oral, pharyngeal and esophageal cancer. *Oral Oncology*, 39 (7), 695-700.

93 Ganmaa, D., Willett, W.C., Li, T.Y., Feskanich, D., van Dam, R.M., Lopez-Garcia, E., Hunter, D.J., Holmes, M.D. (2008) Coffee, tea, caffeine and risk of breast cancer: a 22-year follow-up. *International Journal of Cancer*, 122 (9), 2071-2076.

94 Je, Y., Hankinson, S.E., Tworoger, S.S., Devivo, I., Giovannucci, E. (2011) A prospective cohort study of coffee consumption and risk of endometrial cancer over a 26-year follow-up. *Cancer Epidemiology: Biomarkers & Prevention*, 20 (12), 2487.

95 Harvard Medical School: Harvard Health Publications (2006) *Coffee health benefits – coffee may protect against disease*. [Online]. Available from: http://www.health.harvard.edu/press_releases/coffee_health_benefits. [Accessed 26th July 2012.]

96 Can coffee lower the risk of prostate cancer? Talk of the Nation. National Public Radio. 11th December 2009.

97 MacMahon, (1981) Coffee and cancer of the pancreas. *The New England Journal of Medicine*, 304, 630-633.

98 Jankun, J., Selman, S.H., Swiercz, R., Skrzypczak-Jankun, E. (1997) Why drinking green tea could prevent cancer. *Nature*, 387 (6633), 561.

99 BBC News (2003) Green tea 'can block cancer'. [Online]. Available from: http://news.bbc.co.uk/1/hi/health/3125469.stm [Accessed 4th April 2012.]

100 *The Times* (2007) *Healthy Fellow – Milk and Tea Controversy*. [Online]. Available from: http://www.healthyfellow.com [Accessed 2nd May 2012.]

101 Cancer Research UK. Alcohol and Cancer. [Online]. Available from: http://info.cancerresearchuk.org/healthyliving/alcohol/alcohol-and-cancer [Accessed 2nd May 2012]; Boyle, P., Autier, P., Bartelink, H., Baselga, J., Boffetta, P., Burn, J., Burns, H.J,, Christensen, L., Denis, L., Dicato, M., Diehl, V., Doll, R., Franceschi, S., Gillis, C.R., Gray, N., Griciute, L., Hackshaw, A., Kasler, M., Kogevinas, M., Kvinnsland, S., La Vecchia, C., Levi, F., McVie, J.G., Maisonneuve, P., Martin-Moreno, J.M., Bishop, J.N., Oleari, F., Perrin, P., Quinn, M., Richards, M., Ringborg, U., Scully, C., Siracka, E., Storm, H., Tubiana, M., Tursz, T., Veronesi, U., Wald, N., Weber, W., Zaridze, D. G., Zatonski, W., zur Hausen, H. (2003) European code against cancer and scientific justification: third version. *Annals of Oncology*, 14 (7), 973-1005; IARC (2003) World Cancer Report, ed. B. Stewart and P. Kleihues. Lyon IARC Press; WCRF and AICR (1997) *Food, nutrition and the prevention of cancer: a global perspective*. American Institute for Cancer Research, Washington, 37-145; WHO/FAO (2003) *Joint WHO/FAO Expert Consultation on Diet, Nutrition and the Prevention of Chronic Diseases, in WHO Technical Report Series*. WHO, Geneva. 95-104.

102 Pip, E. (2000) Survey of bottled drinking water available in Manitoba, Canada. *Environmental Health Perspectives*, 108 (9), 863-866.

103 Parkin, M.D., Boyd, L., Walker, L.C. (2011) The fraction of cancer attributable to lifestyle and environmental factors in the UK in 2010. *British Journal of Cancer*, 105, S77-S81.

104 Corrao, G., Bagnardi, V., Zambon, A., La Vecchia, C. (2004) A meta-analysis of alcohol consumption and the risk of 15 diseases. *Preventative Medicine*, 38 (5), 613-619.

105 Key J et al. (2002) Alcohol, tobacco and breast cancer collaborative reanalysis of individual data from 53 epidemiological studies, including 58,515 women with breast cancer and 95,067 women without the disease. *British Journal of Cancer*, 87 (11), 1234-1245; Smith-Warner SA, et al. (1998) Alcohol and breast cancer in women: a pooled analysis of cohort studies. *The Journal of the American Medical Association*, 279, 535-540; Zhang SM, et al. (2007) Alcohol consumption and breast cancer risk in the Women's Health Study. *American Journal of Epidemiology*, 165 (6), 667-676.

106 Harris, H. et al (2012) Alcohol intake and mortality among women with invasive breast cancer. *British journal of Cancer*. 01/05/2012.

107 Pelucchi, C., Galeone, C., Tramacere, I., Bagnardi, V., Negri, E., Islami, F., Scotti, L., Bellocco, R., Corrao, G., Boffetta, P., La Vecchia, C. (2011) *Annals of Oncology*. Advance access published October 29th.

108 Tramacere, I. et al (2011) A meta-analysis on alcohol drinking and gastric cancer risk. *Annals of oncology*, 05/12/2011.

109 Sieja, K., Talerczyk, M. (2004) Selenium as an element in the treatment of ovarian cancer in women receiving chemotherapy. *Gynecologic Oncology*, 93 (2), 320-327; Klein, E., Thompson, I., Tangen, C. et al, Baker, D. (2011) Vitamin E and the risk of prostate cancer. J Amer Med Assoc. Vol. 306, No. 14; Li, K. et al (2011) Vitamin/mineral supplementation and cancer, cardiovascular, and all-cause mortality in a german prospective cohort (EPIC-Heidelberg). European Journal of Nutrition. 07/28/2011.

110 Thomas, D. (2003) A study on the mineral depletion of the foods available to us as a nation over the period 1940 to 1991. *Nutrition and Health*, 17 (2), 85-115.

111 Niki, E., Noguchi, N., Tsuchihashi, H., Gotoh, N. (1995) Interaction among vitamin C, vitamin E and beta-carotene. *The American Journal of Clinical Nutrition*, 62 (6), 1322S-1326S; Winston, C. (2002) *Phytochemicals: guardians of our health*. [Online]. Available from: http://www.andrews. edu/NUFS/phyto. html [Accessed 3rd December 2002.]

112 Campbell, C.T., Campbell, T.M. (2006) *The China Study: the most comprehensive study of nutrition ever conducted and the starting implications for diet, weight loss and long-term health*. Dallas, Texas. BenBella Books.

Step 6 Protect Yourself with Exercise

1 At least five a week: Evidence on the impact of physical activity and its relationship to health. A report by the Chief Medical Officer. Department of Health. 29 April 2004.

2 Ballard-Barbash R, Friedenreich CM, Courneya KS, Siddiqi SM, McTiernan A, Alfano CM (2012) Physical activity, biomarkers, and disease outcomes in cancer survivors: a systematic review. *J Natl Cancer Inst.* Jun 6;104(11):815-40.

3 Awatef M, et al., (2011) Physical activity reduces breast cancer risk: A case–control study in Tunisia. *Cancer Epidemiol.* Dec;35(6):540-4. Epub 2011 Apr 5; Erbach M et al., (2012) Diabetes and the risk for colorectal cancer. *J Diabetes Complications.* Jan-Feb;26(1):50-5; Faul LA, et al. (2011) Relationship of Exercise to Quality of Life in Cancer Patients Beginning

Chemotherapy. *J Pain Symptom Manage.* May;41(5):859-69. Epub 2011 Feb 18; Huy C et al. (2012) Physical activity in a German breast cancer patient cohort: One-year trends and characteristics associated with change in activity level. *Eur J Cancer.* Feb;48(3):297-304; Jones LW, et al. (2012) Prognostic significance of functional capacity and exercise behaviour in patients with metastatic non-small cell lung cancer. *Lung Cancer.* May;76(2):248-52; Keogh JW, et al. (2012) Body Composition, Physical Fitness, Functional Performance, Quality of Life, and Fatigue Benefits of Exercise for Prostate Cancer Patients: A Systematic Review. *J Pain Symptom Manage.* Jan;43(1):96-110; Linkov F, et al. (2012) Longitudinal evaluation of cancer-associated biomarkers before and after weight loss in RENEW study participants: Implications for cancer risk reduction. *Gynecol Oncol.* Apr;125(1):114-9; Lukowski J, et al. (2012) Endometrial cancer survivors' assessment of the benefits of exercise. *Gynecol Oncol.* Mar;124(3):426-30; Modesitt SC, et al. (2012) Morbidly obese women with and without endometrial cancer: Are there differences in measured physical fitness, body composition, or hormones? Gynecol Oncol. Mar;124(3):431-6; Parent MÉ, et al. (2011) Occupational and recreational physical activity during adult life and the risk of cancer among men. *Cancer Epidemiol.* Apr;35(2):151-9; Rogers LQ, et al. (2012) Better exercise adherence after treatment for cancer (BEAT Cancer) study: Rationale, design, and methods. *Contemp Clin Trials.* Jan;33(1):124-37; Sprod LK, et al. (2012) Exercise and cancer treatment symptoms in 408 newly diagnosed older cancer patients. *J Geriatr Oncol.* Apr 1;3(2):90-97; Winters-Stone KM, et al. (2012) The Exercising Together project: Design and recruitment for a randomized, controlled trial to determine the benefits of partnered strength training for couples coping with prostate cancer. *Contemp Clin Trials.* Mar;33(2):342-50.

4   Awatef M, et al. (2011) Physical activity reduces breast cancer risk: A case–control study in Tunisia. *Cancer Epidemiol.* Dec;35(6):540-4. Epub 2011 Apr 5; Erbach M, et al. (2012) Diabetes and the risk for colorectal cancer. *J Diabetes Complications.* Jan-Feb;26(1):50-5; Faul LA, et al. (2011) Relationship of Exercise to Quality of Life in Cancer Patients Beginning Chemotherapy. *J Pain Symptom Manage.* May;41(5):859-69. Epub 2011 Feb 18; Huy C, et al. (2012) Physical activity in a German breast cancer patient cohort: One-year trends and characteristics associated with change in activity level. *Eur J Cancer.* Feb;48(3):297-304; Jones LW, et al. (2012) Prognostic significance of functional capacity and exercise behaviour in patients with metastatic non-small cell lung cancer. *Lung Cancer.* May;76(2):248-52; Keogh JW, et al. (2012) Body Composition, Physical Fitness, Functional Performance, Quality of Life, and Fatigue Benefits of Exercise for Prostate Cancer Patients: A Systematic Review. *J Pain Symptom Manage.* Jan;43(1):96-110; Linkov F, et al. (2012) Longitudinal evaluation of cancer-associated biomarkers before and after weight loss in RENEW study participants: Implications for cancer risk reduction. *Gynecol Oncol.* Apr;125(1):114-9; Lukowski J, et al. (2012) Endometrial cancer survivors' assessment of the benefits of exercise. *Gynecol Oncol.* Mar;124(3):426-30; Modesitt SC, et al. (2012) Morbidly obese women with and without endometrial cancer: Are there differences in measured physical fitness, body composition, or hormones? *Gynecol Oncol.* Mar;124(3):431-6; Parent MÉ, et al. (2011) Occupational and recreational physical activity during adult life and the risk of cancer among men. *Cancer Epidemiol.* Apr;35(2):151-9; Rogers LQ, et al. (2012) Better exercise adherence after treatment for cancer (BEAT Cancer) study: Rationale, design, and methods. *Contemp Clin Trials.* Jan;33(1):124-

37; Sprod LK, et al. (2012) Exercise and cancer treatment symptoms in 408 newly diagnosed older cancer patients. *J Geriatr Oncol.* Apr 1;3(2):90-97; Winters-Stone KM, et al. (2012) The Exercising Together project: Design and recruitment for a randomized, controlled trial to determine the benefits of partnered strength training for couples coping with prostate cancer. *Contemp Clin Trials.* Mar;33(2):342-50.

5   The importance of physical activity for people living with and beyond cancer: A concise evidence review. Macmillan Cancer Support. July 2011.

7   Depledge, M. and Bird, W. (2009) The Blue Gym: Health and wellbeing from our coasts. *Marine Pollution Bulletin.* 58, 947-958; Bird, W. (2005) Walking the way to health. Evidence based Healthcare and Public Health. 9, 171-172; Bird, W. (2004) Can Green Space and Biodiversity increase levels of physical activity? A report for the Royal Society for the Protection of Birds; Bird, W. (2007) Natural Thinking. A report for the Royal Society for the Protection of Birds: Investigating the links between the natural environment, biodiversity and mental health.

8   Bird, W. (2005) Walking the way to health. *Evidence based Healthcare and Public Health.* 9, 171-172.

9   Bird, W. (2004) Can Green Space and Biodiversity increase levels of physical activity? A report for the Royal Society for the Protection of Birds.

10 http://www.walkingforhealth.org.uk

11 Granacher U, Muehlbauer T, Bridenbaugh SA, Wolf M, Roth R, Gschwind Y, Wolf I, Mata R, Kressig RW. (2012) Effects of a Salsa Dance Training on Balance and Strength Performance in Older Adults. *Gerontology.* 2012 Jan 6. [Epub ahead of print.]

12 Kim S, Kim J. (2007) Mood after various brief exercise and sport modes: aerobics, hip-hop dancing, ice skating, and body conditioning. *Percept Mot Skills.* Jun;104(3 Pt 2):1265-70.

13 Sandel SL, Judge JO, Landry N, Faria L, Ouellette R, Majczak M. (2005) Dance and movement program improves quality-of-life measures in breast cancer survivors. *Cancer Nurs.* Jul-Aug;28(4):301-9.

14 Kaltsatou, A., Mameletzi, D., Douka, S. (2011) Physical and psychological benefits of a 24-week traditional dance program in breast cancer survivors. *Journal of Bodywork & Movement Therapies* 15, 162-167.

15 Servan-Schreber, D. (2005) *Healing without Freud or Prozac: Natural Approaches to Curing Stress, Anxiety, Depression without Drugs and without Psychotherapy.* Rodale International Limited.

16 www.macmillan.org.uk

17 At least five a week: Evidence on the impact of physical activity and its relationship to health. A report by the Chief Medical Officer. Department of Health. 29 April 2004.

18 Ballard-Barbash R, Berrigan D, Potischman N, Dowling E. (2010) Obesity and cancer epidemiology. In: Berger NA, editor. *Cancer and Energy Balance, Epidemiology and Overview.* New York: Springer-Verlag New York, LLC; Rao GH, Thethi I, Fareed J.(2011) Vascular disease: obesity and excess weight as modulators of risk. *Expert Rev Cardiovasc Ther.* Apr;9(4):525-34; Lazarou C, Panagiotakos D, Matalas AL (2012) The role of diet in prevention and management of type 2 diabetes: implications for public health. *Crit Rev Food Sci Nutr.* 2012;52(5):382-9.

19 Simpson RJ, Lowder TW, Spielmann G, Bigley AB, Lavoy EC, Kunz H. (2012) Exercise and the aging immune system. *Ageing Res Rev.* Jul;11(3):404-20.

20 Antony GK, Dudek AZ. (2010) Interleukin 2 in cancer therapy. *Curr Med Chem.*17(29):3297-302.

21 At least five a week: Evidence on the impact of physical activity and its relationship to health. A report by the Chief Medical Officer. Department of Health. 29 April 2004; Plant, J., Stephenson, J. (2008) *Beating Stress, Anxiety and Depression*. Piaktus Books.

Step 7 Be Aware of Your Environment

1 http://www.atsdr.cdc.gov/risk/cancer/cancer-introduction.html

2 Rafnsson, V., Hrafnkelsson J., and Tulinius H. (2000). Incidence of cancer among commercial airline pilots. *Occup Environ Med.* 2000 March; 57(3): 175-179.

3 McKinlay, R., Plant, J.A., Bell, J.N. & Voulvoulis N. (2008a) Calculating human exposure to endocrine disrupting pesticides via agricultural and non-agricultural exposure routes. *Science of the Total Environment* 398 (1-3) 1-12; Knopper, L.D. & D.R.S. Lean (2004). Carcinogenic and Genotoxic Potential of Turf Pesticides Commonly Used on Golf Courses. *Journal of Toxicology and Environmental Health*, Part B. 7 267-279.

4 McCarrison, R. (1921) *Studies in Deficiency Disease*. Oxford Medical Publications, Henry Frowde and Hodder & Stoughton, London; Howard, A (1940) An Agricultural Testament. Oxford University Press.

5 European Environment Agency (2001). Environmental Signals 2001. Environmental Assessment Report No. 8. Published May 29, 2001.

6 Carson, R (1962) *Silent Spring*. Penguin Books.

7 UNEP annual report, page 80, http://www.unep.org/pdf/UNEP_ANNUAL_REPORT_2012.pdf.

8 Reducing Environmental Cancer Risk: What We Can Do Now. 2008-2009 Annual Report by the Presidents Cancer Panel. Published April 2010.

9 Environmental Protection Agency. EPA regulations (40 CFR Sec. 156.10).

10 Reducing Environmental Cancer Risk: What We Can Do Now. 2008-2009 Annual Report by the Presidents Cancer Panel. Published April 2010.

11 The impacts of endocrine disrupters on wildlife, people and their environments – The Weybridge+15 (1996–2011) report. EEA (European Environment Agency). Published: May 10, 2012.

12 Colborn, T., Dumanoski, D., Meyers, J. (1997). *Our Stolen Future : How We Are Threatening Our Fertility, Intelligence and Survival*. Plume.

13 McKinlay R, Dassyne J, Djamgoz MBA, Plant JA, Voulvoulis N (2012) Agricultural pesticides and chemical fertilisers. In *Pollutants, Human Health and the Environment: A risk based approach*. Wiley-Blackwell Publishers.

14 McKinlay R, Dassyne J, Djamgoz MBA, Plant JA, Voulvoulis N (2012) Agricultural pesticides and chemical fertilisers. In *Pollutants, Human Health and the Environment: A risk based approach*. Wiley-Blackwell Publishers.

15 McDuffie HH. (2005) Host factors and genetic susceptibility: a paradigm of the conundrum of pesticide exposure and cancer associations. *Rev Environ Health.* Apr-Jun;20(2):77-101.

16 Skakkebak NE, Rajpert-De Meyts E, Main KM (2001). Testicular dysgenesis syndrome: An increasingly common developmental disorder with environmental aspects. *Opinion. Hum Reprod.* 16:972-978.

17 Keri R, Ho SM, Hunt PA, Knudsen KE, Soto AM & Prins GS (2007) An evaluation of evidence for the carcinogenic activity of bisphenol A: report of NIEHS Expert Panel on BPA. *Reproductive Toxicology* 24, 240-252.

18 Herbst AL, Ulfelder H, Poskanzer DC. (1971) Adenocarcinoma of the vagina. Association of maternal stilbestrol therapy with tumor appearance in young women. *N Engl J Med.* Apr 15;284(15):878-81.

19 Darbre PD. (2006) Environmental oestrogens, cosmetics and breast cancer. *Best Pract Res Clin Endocrinol Metab.* Mar;20(1):121-43; Fenton SE. (2006) Endocrine-disrupting compounds and mammary gland development: early exposure and later life consequences. *Endocrinology.* Jun;147(6 Suppl):S18-24.

20 Royal Commission on Environmental Pollution (2003) Chemicals in Products – Safeguarding the Environment and Human Health Cm 5827, 24th report, June 2003.

21 Hutchings et al. (2012) Occupational cancer in Britain. Industry sector results. Hutchings SJ, Rushton L; British Occupational Cancer Burden Study Group. *Br J Cancer.* 2012 Jun 19;107 Suppl 1:S92-S103.

22 Cadogan David F. and Howick Christopher J. (2000) Plasticizers, In *Ullmann's Encyclopedia of Industrial Chemistry*, Wiley-VCH, Weinheim.

23 Barrett JR. (2005) The ugly side of beauty products. *Environ Health Perspect.* Jan;113(1):A24; Rudel RA, Perovich LJ. (2009) Endocrine disrupting chemicals in indoor and outdoor air. *Atmos Environ.* 2009 Jan 1;43(1):170-181.

24 Hernández-Díaz S, Mitchell AA, Kelley KE, Calafat AM, Hauser R (2009). Medications as a potential source of exposure to phthalates in the U.S. population. *Environ Health Perspec*t. Feb;117(2):185-9.

25 Meeker JD, Calafat AM, Hauser R (2009) Urinary metabolites of di(2-ethylhexyl) phthalate are associated with decreased steroid hormone levels in adult men. *J Androl.* 2009 May-Jun;30(3):287-97.

26 Swan SH. (2008) Environmental phthalate exposure in relation to reproductive outcomes and other health endpoints in humans. *Environ Res.* Oct;108(2):177-84; Virtanen HE, Rajpert-De Meyts E, Main KM, Skakkebaek NE, Toppari J. (2005) Testicular dysgenesis syndrome and the development and occurrence of male reproductive disorders. *Toxicol Appl Pharmacol.* Sep 1;207(2 Suppl):501-5.

27 Rubin BS. (2011) Bisphenol A: an endocrine disruptor with widespread exposure and multiple effects. *J Steroid Biochem Mol Biol.* Oct;127(1-2):27-34.

28 http://www.time.com/time/specials/packages/article/0,28804,1976909_1976908_1976938,00.html

29 Bisphenol A (BPA) – Current state of knowledge and future actions by WHO and FAO; 27 November 2009.

30 Soto, A.M., Sonnenschein, C. (2010). Environmental causes of cancer: endocrine disruptors as carcinogens. *Nature Reviews Endocrinology* 6 (7): 363-370.

31 Brisken, C. (2008). Endocrine Disruptors and Breast Cancer. *CHIMIA International Journal for Chemistry* 62 (5): 406–409; Soto, A.; Vandenberg, L.; Maffini, M.; Sonnenschein, C. (2008). Does breast cancer start in the womb? *Basic & Clinical Pharmacology & Toxicology* 102 (2): 125-133; Fernandez, S. V. Russo, J. (2009). Estrogen and Xenoestrogens in Breast Cancer. *Toxicologic Pathology* 38 (1): 110-122; Jenkins, S.; Raghuraman, N.; Eltoum, I.; Carpenter, M.; Russo, J.; Lamartiniere, C.A. (2009). Oral Exposure to Bisphenol A Increases Dimethylbenzanthracene-Induced Mammary Cancer in Rats (Free full text). *Environmental Health Perspectives* 117 (6): 910-915; Betancourt, A.; Mobley, J.; Russo, J.; Lamartiniere, C. (2010). Proteomic Analysis in Mammary Glands of Rat Offspring Exposed In Utero to Bisphenol A. *Journal of proteomics* 73 (6): 1241-1253.

32 Nagel, S.C.; Vom Saal, F.S.; Thayer, K.A.; Dhar, M.G.; Boechler, M.; Welshons, W. V. (1997). Relative binding affinity-serum modified access (RBA-SMA)

assay predicts the relative in vivo bioactivity of the xenoestrogens bisphenol A and octylphenol. *Environmental health perspectives* (Brogan & Partners) 105 (1): 70-76; Timms, B.; Howdeshell, K.; Barton, L.; Bradley, S.; Richter, C.; Vom Saal, F. (2005). Estrogenic chemicals in plastic and oral contraceptives disrupt development of the fetal mouse prostate and urethra. *Proceedings of the National Academy of Sciences of the United States of America* 102 (19): 7014-7019; Ho, S.; Tang, W.; Belmonte De Frausto, J.; Prins, G. (2006). Developmental exposure to estradiol and bisphenol a increases susceptibility to prostate carcinogenesis and epigenetically regulates phosphodiesterase type 4 variant 4. *Cancer Research* 66 (11): 5624-5632; Richter, C.; Taylor, J.; Ruhlen, R.; Welshons, W.; Vom Saal, F. (2007). Estradiol and Bisphenol a stimulate androgen receptor and estrogen receptor gene expression in fetal mouse prostate mesenchyme cells. *Environmental health perspectives* 115 (6): 902-908; Prins, G.; Tang, W.; Belmonte, J.; Ho, S. (2008). Developmental exposure to bisphenol a increases prostate cancer susceptibility in adult rats: epigenetic mode of action is implicated. *Fertility and Sterility* 89 (2 Suppl): e41-e41.

33 Zhu, H.; Xiao, X.; Zheng, J.; Zheng, S.; Dong, K.; Yu, Y. (2009). Growth-promoting effect of bisphenol a on neuroblastoma in vitro and in vivo. *Journal of Pediatric Surgery* 44 (4): 672-680; Zheng, J.; Xiao, X.; Liu, J.; Zheng, S.; Yin, Q.; Yu, Y. (2007). Growth-promoting effect of environmental endocrine disruptors on human neuroblastoma SK-N-SH cells. *Environmental Toxicology and Pharmacology* 24 (2): 189-193; Zhu, H.; Zheng, J.; Xiao, X.; Zheng, S.; Dong, K.; Liu, J.; Wang, Y. (2010). Environmental endocrine disruptors promote invasion and metastasis of SK-N-SH human neuroblastoma cells. *Oncology reports* 23 (1): 129-139; Reducing Environmental Cancer Risk: What We Can Do Now. 2008-2009 Annual Report by the Presidents Cancer Panel. Published April 2010.

34 Reducing Environmental Cancer Risk: What We Can Do Now. 2008-2009 Annual Report by the Presidents Cancer Panel. Published April 2010.

35 Brody JG, Maysich KB, Humblet O, Attfield KR, Beehler GP, Rudel RA. Environmental pollutants and breast cancer: epidemiologic studies. *Cancer.* 2007;109(12 Suppl):2667-711.

36 Prince MM, Ruder AM, Hein MJ, Waters MA, Whelan EA, Nilsen N, et al. (2006) Mortality and exposure response among 14,458 electrical capacitor manufacturing workers exposed to polychlorinated biphenyls (PCBs). *Environ Health Perspect.* 114(1):1508-14.

37 Ruder AM, Hein MJ, Nilsen N, Waters MA, Laber P, Davis-King K, et al. (2006) Mortality among workers exposed to polychlorinated biphenyls (PCBs) in an electrical capacitor manufacturing plant in Indiana: an update. *Environ Health Perspect.* 114(1):18-23.

38 http://en.wikipedia.org/wiki/polychlorinated_biphenyl

39 Ohandja D-G, Donovan S, Castle P, Voulvoulis N, Plant JA (2012) Regulatory systems and guidelines for the management of risk. In *Pollutants, Human Health and the Environment: A risk based approach.* Wiley-Blackwell Publishers.

40 McKinlay R, Dassyne J, Djamgoz MBA, Plant JA, Voulvoulis N (2012) Agricultural pesticides and chemical fertilisers. In *Pollutants, Human Health and the Environment: A risk based approach.* Wiley-Blackwell Publishers.

41 International Agency for Research on Cancer (IARC) Monograph Vol. 5, 30 and 53.

42 Environment Agency (1998) Endocrine – disrupting substances in the Environment: what should be done? Consultation paper; ENDS (1999),

Industry glimpses new challenges as endocrine science advances. ENDS Report 290: 26-30.

43 http://www.pan-uk.org/pestnews/Actives/endocrin.htm

44 http://articles.latimes.com/2011/aug/31/local/la-me-pesticides-cancer-20110831

45 Lowengart, R. et al., (1987) Childhood Leukemia and Parent's Occupational and Home Exposures, *Journal of the National Cancer Institute* 79:39.

46 Lu JL.(2005) Risk factors to pesticide exposure and associated health symptoms among cut-flower farmers. *Int J Environ Health Res.* Jun;15(3):161-9; Lu JL. (2007) Acute pesticide poisoning among cut-flower farmers. J Environ Health. Sep;70(2):38-43.

47 Menegaux F, Baruchel A, Bertrand Y, Lescoeur B, Leverger G, Nelken B, Sommelet D, Hémon D, Clavel J (2006) Household exposure to pesticides and risk of childhood acute leukaemia. *Occup Environ Med.* Feb;63(2):131-4.

48 The Royal Commission on Environmental Pollution (RCEP) (2005) Crop spraying and the Health of Residents and Bystanders. Report.

49 Davis BN, Brown MJ, Frost AJ, Yates TJ, Plant JA (1994) The effects of hedges on spray deposition and on the biological impact of pesticide spray drift. *Ecotoxicol Environ Saf.* Apr;27(3):281-93.

50 Valcke M, Samuel O, Bouchard M, Dumas P, Belleville D, Tremblay C.(2006) Biological monitoring of exposure to organophosphate pesticides in children living in peri-urban areas of the Province of Quebec, Canada. *Int Arch Occup Environ Health.* Aug;79(7):568-77; Li XH, Wang W, Wang J, Cao XL, Wang XF, Liu JC, Liu XF, Xu XB, Jiang XN.(2008) Contamination of soils with organochlorine pesticides in urban parks in Beijing, China. *Chemosphere.* Feb;70(9):1660-8. Epub 2007 Sep 14.

51 Rayman RB. (2006) Aircraft disinfection. *Aviat Space Environ Med.* Jul;77(7):733-6; Sutton PM, Vergara X, Beckman J, Nicas M, Das R. (2007) Pesticide illness among flight attendants due to aircraft disinsection. *Am J Ind Med.* May;50(5):345-56.

52 Kross BC, Burmeister LF, Ogilvie LK, Fuortes LJ, Fu CM. (1996) Proportionate mortality study of golf course superintendents. *Am J Ind Med.* May;29(5):501-6.

53 Lithner, D. (2011) Environmental and health hazards of chemicals in plastic polymers and products. Department of Plant and Environmental Sciences University of Gothenburg. Thesis was successfully defended in public on 6 May 2011.

54 http://www.sciencedaily.com/releases/2009/08/090819234651.htm

55 Lithner, D. (2011) Environmental and health hazards of chemicals in plastic polymers and products. Department of Plant and Environmental Sciences University of Gothenburg. Thesis was successfully defended in public on 6 May 2011.

56 Braungart, M. (2008) Cradle to Cradle design – 'Beyond Reach'. Lecture given at the UK Chemical Stakeholder Forum. London, June 20, 2008.

57 Muncke J. (2011) Endocrine disrupting chemicals and other substances of concern in food contact materials: an updated review of exposure, effect and risk assessment. *J Steroid Biochem Mol Biol.* Oct;127(1-2):118-27.

58 Wagner M, Oehlmann J. (2011) Endocrine disruptors in bottled mineral water: estrogenic activity in the E-Screen. *J Steroid Biochem Mol Biol.* Oct;127(1-2):128-35.

59 Braungart, M. (2008) Cradle to Cradle design – 'Beyond Reach'. Lecture given at the UK Chemical Stakeholder Forum. London, June 20, 2008.

60 http://www.fda.gov/Cosmetics/default.htm

61 Brody JG, Maysich KB, Humblet O, Attfield KR, Beehler GP, Rudel RA. (2007) Environmental pollutants and breast cancer: epidemiologic studies. *Cancer.* 109(12 Suppl):2667-711.

62 http://www.marketresearch.com/PharmaLive-Special-Reports-v3422/Appliance-Statistical-Review-2749810/

63 The impacts of endocrine disrupters on wildlife, people and their environments – The Weybridge+15 (1996–2011) report. EEA (European Environment Agency). Published: May 10, 2012.

64 Barrett JR. (2005) The ugly side of beauty products. *Environ Health Perspect.* Jan;113(1):A24.

65 Darbre PD, Aljarrah A, Miller WR, Coldham NG, Sauer MJ, Pope GS (2004). Concentrations of parabens in human breast tumours. *J Appl Toxicol.* Jan-Feb;24(1):5-13.

66 The impacts of endocrine disrupters on wildlife, people and their environments – The Weybridge+15 (1996–2011) report. EEA (European Environment Agency). Published: May 10, 2012.

67 http://www.fda.gov/NewsEvents/Newsroom/PressAnnouncements/ucm258940.htm

68 Consumer Protection. Environmental protection, health and safety. The REACH Enforcement Regulations 2008. 2008 No. 2852.

69 http://www.thedailygreen.com/environmental-news/latest/perfume-chemicals-toxic-0525#ixzz1yz9pyWNy

70 International Agency for Research on Cancer, Monograph Vol. 57 (1993) (p. 43).

71 Braungart, M. (2008) Cradle to Cradle design – 'Beyond Reach'. Lecture given at the UK Chemical Stakeholder Forum. London, June 20, 2008.

72 NCRP Report No. 160 on increased average radiation exposure of the US population. Public release date: 3-Mar-2009.

73 http://www.bloomberg.com/news/2011-09-12/commonly-used-pain-pills-increase-kidney-cancer-risk-in-study.html

74 Hernández-Díaz S, Mitchell AA, Kelley KE, Calafat AM, Hauser R (2009). Medications as a potential source of exposure to phthalates in the U.S. population. *Environ Health Perspect.* Feb;117(2):185-9.

75 Golding SJ, Shrimpton PC.(2002) Commentary. Radiation dose in CT: are we meeting the challenge? *Br J Radiol.* Jan;75(889):1-4; Brenner DJ, Hall EJ.(2007) Computed tomography--an increasing source of radiation exposure. *N Engl J Med.* Nov 29;357(22):2277-84.

76 Hardell L, Carlberg M. (2009) Mobile phones, cordless phones and the risk for brain tumours. *Int J Oncol.* Jul;35(1):5-17; Yakymenko I, Sidorik E (2010) Risks of carcinogenesis from electromagnetic radiation of mobile telephony devices. *Exp Oncol.* Jul;32(2):54-60; Yakymenko I, Sidorik E, Kyrylenko S, Chekhun V (2011) Long-term exposure to microwave radiation provokes cancer growth: evidences from radars and mobile communication systems. *Exp Oncol.* Jun;33(2):62-70; Lehrer S, Green S, Stock RG. (2011) Association between number of cell phone contracts and brain tumor incidence in nineteen U.S. States. *J Neurooncol.* Feb;101(3):505-7.

77 Baan R, Grosse Y, Lauby-Secretan B, El Ghissassi F, Bouvard V, Benbrahim-Tallaa L, Guha N, Islami F, Galichet L, Straif K; WHO International Agency for Research on Cancer Monograph Working Group. Carcinogenicity of radiofrequency electromagnetic fields. *Lancet Oncol.* 2011 Jul;12(7):624-6; . http://monographs.iarc.fr/ENG/Monographs/PDFs/index.php Monograph no. 102.

78 Agency for Toxic Substances and Disease Registry (2008). ToxFAQ for Radon. September 2008.

79 Gray A, Read S, McGale P, Darby S. (2009) Lung cancer deaths from indoor radon and the cost effectiveness and potential of policies to reduce them. *BMJ* Jan 6;338:a3110. doi: 10.1136/bmj.a3110.77.

80 A Citizen's Guide to Radon. United States Environmental Protection Agency. October 12, 2010. http://www.epa.gov/radon/pubs/citguide.html

81 Joint FAO/WHO Expert Committee on Food Additives (1983). *Evaluation of certain food additives and contaminants.* Geneva, World Health Organization. Twenty-seventh report, (WHO Technical Report Series, No. 696).

82 Plant J., Voulvoulis, N., Ragnarsdottir, K. (2012) *Pollutants, Human Health and the Environment: A risk based approach.* Wiley-Blackwell Publishers.

83 www.bgs.ac.uk

84 Waalkes MP, Liu J, Diwan BA. (2007). Transplacental arsenic carcinogenesis in mice. *Toxicology and Applied Pharmacology* 222:271–280.

85 Xu Y, Tokar EJ, Sun Y, Waalkes MP (2012). Arsenic-Transformed Malignant Prostate Epithelia Can Convert Noncontiguous Normal Stem Cells into an Oncogenic Phenotype. *Environmental Health Perspectives.* 120:865-871.

86 Smith AH, Steinmaus CM(2000). Arsenic in urine and drinking water. *Environ Health Perspect.* Nov;108(11):A494-5.

87 Hall AH (2002). Chronic arsenic poisoning. *Toxicol Lett.* Mar 10;128(1-3):69-72; Tseng CH, Tseng CP, Chiou HY, Hsueh YM, Chong CK, Chen CJ (2002) Epidemiologic evidence of diabetogenic effect of arsenic. *Toxicol Lett.* Jul 7;133(1):69-76.

88 Ng JC, Wang J, Shraim A (2003). A global health problem caused by arsenic from natural sources. Chemosphere. Sep;52(9):1353-9.

89 Mercer TG, Frostick LE. Leaching characteristics of CCA-treated wood waste: a UK study. *Sci Total Environ.* 2012 Jun 15;427-428:165-74. Epub 2012 May 8.

90 Steinemann, A.C. (2009). Fragranced consumer products and undisclosed ingredients. *Environmental Impact Assessment Review*, 29, 32-38.

91 http://www.epa.gov/iaq/pubs/insidestory.html

92 http://www.preventcancer.com/consumers/household/carcinogens_home.htm

93 Goldberg MS, Siemiatyck J, DeWar R, Désy M, Riberdy H (1999) Risks of developing cancer relative to living near a municipal solid waste landfill site in Montreal, Quebec, Canada. *Arch Environ Health.* Jul-Aug;54(4):291-6.

94 Knox, EG. (2000) Childhood cancers, birthplaces, incinerators and landfill sites. *International Journal of Epidemiology.* 29: 391-397; Jarup L, Briggs D, de Hoogh C, Morris S, Hurt C, Lewin A, Maitland I, Richardson S, Wakefield J, Elliott P. (2002) Cancer risks in populations living near landfill sites in Great Britain. *Br J Cancer.* Jun 5;86(11):1732-6.

95 Minichilli F, Bartolacci S, Buiatti E, Pallante V, Scala D, Bianchi F (2005) [A study on mortality around six municipal solid waste landfills in Tuscany Region.] *Epidemiol Prev.*Sep-Dec;29(5-6 Suppl):53-6.

96 Porta D, Milani S, Lazzarino AI, Perucci CA, Forastiere F (2009) Systematic review of epidemiological studies on health effects associated with management of solid waste. *Environ Health.* 2009 Dec 23;8:60; Gouveia N, Prado RR. (2010) Health risks in areas close to urban solid waste landfill sites. *Rev Saude Publica.* 2010 Oct;44(5):859-66. Epub 2010 Sep 3.

97 Rapiti E, Sperati A, Fano V, Dell'Orco V (1997) Forastiere FMortality among workers at municipal waste incinerators in Rome: a retrospective cohort study. *Am J Ind Med.* May;31(5):659-61.

98 Elliott P, Eaton N, Shaddick G, Carter R (2000). Cancer incidence near municipal solid waste incinerators in Great Britain. Part 2: histopathological and case-note review of primary liver cancer cases. *Br J Cancer.* Mar;82(5):1103-6.
99 Knox, EG. (2000) Childhood cancers, birthplaces, incinerators and landfill sites. *International Journal of Epidemiology.* 29: 391-397; Floret N, Mauny F, Challier B, Arveux P, Cahn JY, Viel JF (2003) Dioxin emissions from a solid waste incinerator and risk of non-Hodgkin lymphoma. *Epidemiology.* Jul;14(4):392-8; Zambon P, Ricci P, Bovo E, Casula A, Gattolin M, Fiore AR, Chiosi F, Guzzinati S (2007). Sarcoma risk and dioxin emissions from incinerators and industrial plants: a population-based case-control study (Italy). *Environ Health.* Jul 16;6:19.
100 Viel JF, Daniau C, Goria S, Fabre P, de Crouy-Chanel P, Sauleau EA, Empereur-Bissonnet P. (2008) Risk for non Hodgkin's lymphoma in the vicinity of French municipal solid waste incinerators. *Environ Health.* Oct 29;7:51; Viel JF, Floret N, Deconinck E, Focant JF, De Pauw E, Cahn JY. (2011) Increased risk of non-Hodgkin lymphoma and serum organochlorine concentrations among neighbors of a municipal solid waste incinerator. *Environ Int.* Feb;37(2):449-53.
101 Ranzi A, Fano V, Erspamer L, Lauriola P, Perucci CA, Forastiere F. (2011) Mortality and morbidity among people living close to incinerators: a cohort study based on dispersion modelling for exposure assessment. *Environ Health.* Mar 24;10:22.

Step 8 Manage Stress

1 Plant, Jane, 2007. *Your Life in Your Hands.* Fourth edition. Virgin Books.
2 Selye, H., 1936. A syndrome produced by diverse nocuous agents. *Nature,* 138, 32; Selye, H., 1946. The general adaptation syndrome and the diseases of adaptation. *The Journal of Clinical Endocrinology & Metabolism,* 6 (2), 117-230; Selye, H., 1950. Stress and the general adaptation syndrome. *British Medical Journal,* 4667, 1383-1392; Selye, H., 1975. Stress and distress. *Comprehensive Therapy,* 1 (8), 9-13.
3 Lechin, F., van der Dijs, B., Lechin, M. E., 2002. *Neurocircuitry and Neuroautonomic Disorders – Reviews and Therapeutic Strategies.* Karger.
4 Lechin, F., van der Dijs, B., Lechin, M. E., 2002. *Neurocircuitry and Neuroautonomic Disorders – Reviews and Therapeutic Strategies.* Karger; Plant, Jane and Stephenson, Janet, 2011. *Beating Stress, Anxiety and Depression.* Reprint edition. Piatkus.
5 Jen-Chieh Chuang, Mario Perello, Ichiro Sakata, Sherri Osborne-Lawrence, Joseph M Savitt, Michael Lutter, and Jeffrey M Zigman, 2011. Ghrelin mediates stress-induced food-reward behavior in mice. *J Clin Invest.* 2011 July 1; 121(7): 2684-2692, Published online 2011 June 23. doi: 10.1172/JCI57660 PMCID: PMC3223843.
6 Kandel, E.R., Schwartz, J.H., Jessell, T.M., 2000. *Principles of Neural Science.* 4th Edition. USA, McGraw-Hill.
7 White, C.A. and Macleod, U., 2002. ABC of psychological medicine – cancer. *British Medical Journal,* 325, 377-380.
8 APPGITA – All Party Parliamentary Group for Involuntary Tranquilliser Addiction, 2008. Proposals for Manifesto from APPG on Involuntary Tranquilliser Addiction. www.benzo.org.uk/appg2.htm
9 www.cancersupportinternational.com
10 Epel, E.S., Lin, J., Dhabhar, F.S., Wolkowitz, O.M., Puterman, E., Karan, L. and Blackburn, E., 2010. Dynamics of telomerase activity in response to acute psychological stress. *Brain, Behaviour and Immunity,* 24, 531-539.

11 Plant, Jane and Stephenson, Janet, 2011. *Beating Stress, Anxiety and Depression*. Reprint edition. Piatkus.

12 Folkman, S. and Lazarus, R.S., 1988. The relationship between coping and emotion: Implications for theory and research. *Social Science & Medicine*, 26 (3), 309-317.

13 Plant, Jane and Stephenson, Janet, 2011. *Beating Stress, Anxiety and Depression*. Reprint edition. Piatkus.

14 www.volunteering.org.uk

15 Mars, T.S., Abbey, H., 2010. Mindfulness meditation practice as a healthcare intervention: A systematic review. *International Journal of Osteopathic Medicine*, 13, 56-66.

16 Servan-Schreiber, D., 2005. *Healing without Freud or Prozac: Natural approaches to curing stress, anxiety and depression*. Revised edition. London, Rodale Publishing Ltd.

17 Depledge, M.H. and Bird, W.J., 2009. The blue gym: Health and wellbeing from our coasts. *Marine Pollution Bulletin*, 58, 947-948.

Step 9 Broaden Your Awareness

1 Forbes business information, February 2012, http://www.forbes.com/sites/matthewherper/2012/02/10/the-truly-staggering-cost-of-inventing-new-drugs/

2 http://www.pinkribbon.org/About/History/tabid/199/Default.aspx

3 Breast Cancer: An environmental disease (2005), http://www.nomorebreastcancer.org.uk/introduction.html

4 http://www.worldcancerday.org/press-release-wcd-2014

5 Epstein, S.S., 2011. *NATIONAL CANCER INSTITUTE and AMERICAN CANCER SOCIETY Criminal Indifference to Cancer Prevention and Conflicts of Interest*. Xlibris, Corp.

Step 10 Stay on Course

1 Ornish D., Weidner, G., Fair, W.R., Marlin, R., Pettengill, E.B., Raisin, C.J., et al., (2005) Intensive lifestyle changes may affect the progression of prostate cancer. *Journal Of Urology*, 174 (3), 1065-1069; Parasramka MA, Dashwood WM, Wang R, Abdelli A, Bailey GS, Williams DE, Ho E, Dashwood RH. (2012) MicroRNA profiling of carcinogen-induced rat colon tumors and the influence of dietary spinach. *Mol Nutr Food Res*. 2012 Aug;56(8):1259-69.

2 Downloadable from macmillan.org.uk/Documents/GetInvolved/Campaigns/WorkingThroughCancer/WorkItOut/WorkItOut.pdf

index